Rap. ssessment of
the . ely Ill Patient

The *Essential Clinical Skills for Nurses* series focuses on key clinical skills for nurses and other health professionals. These concise, accessible books assume no prior knowledge and focus on core clinical skills, clearly presenting common clinical procedures and their rationale, together with the essential background theory. Their user-friendly format makes them an indispensable guide to clinical practice for all nurses, especially to student nurses and newly qualified staff.

Other titles in the *Essential Clinical Skills for Nurses* series:

Central Venous Access Devices
Lisa Dougherty
ISBN: 9781405119528

Clinical Assessment and Monitoring in Children
Diana Fergusson
ISBN: 9781405133388

Intravenous Therapy
Theresa Finlay
ISBN: 9780632064519

Respiratory Care
Caia Francis
ISBN: 9781405117173

Care of the Neurological Patient
Helen Iggulden
ISBN: 9781405117166

ECGs for Nurses
Second Edition
Phil Jevon
ISBN: 9781405181624

Monitoring the Critically Ill Patient
Second Edition
Phil Jevon and Beverley Ewens
ISBN: 9781405144407

Treating the Critically Ill Patient
Phil Jevon
ISBN: 9781405141727

Pain Management
Eileen Mann and Eloise Carr
ISBN: 9781405130714

Leg Ulcer Management
Christine Moffatt, Ruth Martin and Rachael Smithdale
ISBN: 9781405134767

Pressure Area Care
Edited by Karen Ousey
ISBN: 9781405112253

Infection Prevention and Control
Christine Perry
ISBN: 9781405140386

Stoma Care
Theresa Porrett and Anthony McGrath
ISBN: 9781405114073

Caring for the Perioperative Patient
Paul Wicker and Joy O'Neill
ISBN: 9781405128025

Nursing Medical Emergency Patients
Philip Jevon, Melanie Humphreys and Beverley Ewens
ISBN: 9781405120555

Wound Management
Carol Dealey and Janice Cameron
ISBN: 9781405155410

Trauma Care
Elaine Cole
ISBN: 9781405162302

Clinical Examination Skills
Phil Jevon
ISBN: 9781405178860

Care of the Dying and Dead Patient
Phil Jevon
ISBN: 9781405183390

Sexual Health
Kathy French
ISBN: 9781405168311

Rapid Assessment of the Acutely Ill Patient

Sheila Adam, RN, BNurs, MSc Nurs
Head of Nursing,
University College London Hospitals
NHS Foundation Trust

Mandy Odell, RN, MA
Consultant Nurse, Critical Care,
Royal Berkshire NHS Foundation Trust

John Welch, RN, BSc (Hons) Psych, MSc Nurs
Nurse Consultant, Critical Care,
University College London Hospitals
NHS Foundation Trust

WILEY-BLACKWELL

A John Wiley & Sons, Ltd., Publication

Blackwell Publishing was acquired by John Wiley & Sons in February 2007.
Blackwell's publishing programme has been merged with Wiley's global
Scientific, Technical, and Medical business to form Wiley-Blackwell.

Registered office
John Wiley & Sons Ltd, The Atrium, Southern Gate, Chichester,
West Sussex, PO19 8SQ, United Kingdom

Editorial offices
9600 Garsington Road, Oxford, OX4 2DQ, United Kingdom
2121 State Avenue, Ames, Iowa 50014-8300, USA

For details of our global editorial offices, for customer services and
for information about how to apply for permission to reuse the
copyright material in this book please see our website at
www.wiley.com/wiley-blackwell.

Library of Congress Cataloging-in-Publication Data

Welch, John, 1960–
Rapid assessment of the acutely ill patient / John Welch, Mandy Odell,
Sheila Adam.
p. ; cm. – (Essential clinical skills for nurses)
Includes bibliographical references and index.
ISBN 978-1-4051-6993-6 (pbk. : alk. paper) 1. Nursing
assessment. 2. Intensive care nursing. I. Odell, Mandy. II. Adam,
Sheila K. III. Title. IV. Series: Essential clinical skills for nurses.
[DNLM: 1. Emergencies–nursing. 2. Acute Disease–nursing.
3. Nursing Assessment. 4. Nursing Care–methods. WY 154 W439r 2010]

RT48.W45 2010
616.07′5–dc22
2009019842

A catalogue record for this book is available from the British Library.

Set in 9 on 11 pt Palatino by
Toppan Best-set Premedia Limited
Printed and bound in Malaysia by KHL Printing Co Sdn Bhd
1   2010

Contents

Foreword

The early recognition and treatment of illness is a fundamental cornerstone of medicine. There are few, if any, serious diseases for which delays in the identification of patient deterioration and its management lead to an improved outcome. Despite this, much of the management of disease has been on the goal of ascertaining a diagnosis, sometimes at the expense of inadvertent inattention to a patient's underlying failing physiology. In some cases this has led to the potentially preventable death of the patient; in others, the patient has suffered organ failure leading to unnecessary intensive care admission and hospital length of stay.

The underlying system errors that contribute to a failure to recognise or respond to patient deterioration have multifactorial origins. However, in most cases, they can be categorised as a failure of ward staff to observe and monitor patients closely and frequently, a failure to recognise the signs of patient deterioration and a failure to call for help. Although not a focus of this book, a failure of response teams to respond can also contribute. It is clear that these problems are not unique to any particular country or healthcare system, as similar issues have been identified in North America, the United Kingdom, mainland Europe, Scandinavia and Australia.

The authors of this book have addressed these issues in a text that gives clear, concise information in a logical order using simple diagrams and icons. They commence with a lucid justification for the need for rapid assessment of the acutely ill ward patient and this is followed by a chapter describing current thinking on rapid response systems and their components. The remainder of the book is focused on the use of a simple, easily reproducible scheme of patient assessment, supplemented where necessary with descriptions of underlining anatomy and physiology, and technical skills.

The authors are respected experts in their field. All are experienced in caring for sick patients in critical care units and in general hospital wards, and assisting general wards staff of all backgrounds, grades and experience in managing sick patient outside the walls of a critical care unit. Nurses and other healthcare professional reading this book, and the patients for whom they care, will benefit immensely from the authors' knowledge and experience.

Gary B Smith, BM, FRCA, FRCP,
Professor,
Portsmouth Hospitals NHS Trust &
the University of Bournemouth,
United Kingdom

Preface

Nurses and other healthcare professionals are caring for more and more patients with potential or actual critical illness on general wards. The key to improved outcomes for these patients is early recognition of deterioration, with prompt and appropriate interventions from competent staff.

This book is a guide for nurses and allied health professionals working in general wards. It explains the important physiological processes underpinning vital body functions, and sets out a structured approach to rapid patient assessment, detailing, in turn, the issues of airway patency, and potential problems with breathing, circulation, and consciousness. The assessment process is completed by a review of everything else that should be considered, a discussion of how patient problems can be communicated most effectively, and how the ward team can work together to deliver patient-centred care. This provides a framework that enables the practitioner to obtain and interpret essential data from clinical examination and laboratory results in an ordered fashion that highlights the priorities of care. Signs and symptoms of common problems are described, and fundamental treatments applicable to all serious illnesses are outlined with real-life patient cases used to help the reader apply theory to practice situations.

The authors have many years' experience leading critical care outreach services working with ward staff caring for deteriorating patients. They have written this book in order to share their accumulated knowledge and skills so that seriously ill patients may benefit – wherever they are cared for.

Why Rapid Assessment Is Essential for Ward Staff

INTRODUCTION

There is an increasing emphasis in the modern health service on managing most illnesses in community settings and performing most surgery in day surgery units. Consequently, the number of inpatient beds has fallen by about 40% in the past 25 years, although in the same period numbers of hospital admissions have risen by 74% (NHS Confederation, 2006; Hospital Episode Statistics inpatient data, 2006–07). In addition, an increasing proportion of patients are admitted as emergencies: there were 4.7 million emergency admissions in 2006–2007, equating to 36% of all in-patient cases (Hospital Episode Statistics inpatient data, 2006–07). Therefore, hospital occupancy and throughput rates are generally high, and the relative numbers of acutely and critically ill patients have significantly increased. Furthermore, the proportion of older patients in hospital is also rising each year: 41% of adult inpatients were aged 65 years or more in 2006–2007 (Hospital Episode Statistics inpatient data, 2006–07), and this group often have one or more chronic conditions that increase the complexity of their care.

Factors contributing to increased acuity of general ward patients are:

- Faster throughput
- Increased numbers of emergency cases – more acute and critical illness
- Increased numbers of older patients – more complex, chronic disease
- More aggressive and invasive treatments.

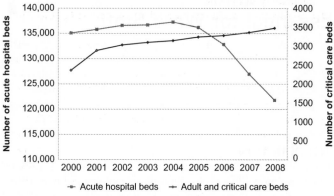

Number of acute and critical care beds in England 2000-2008

Fig. 1.1 Numbers of all acute care beds and critical care beds in England 2000–2008
Sources: www.performance.doh.gov.uk/hospitalactivity/data_requests/download/beds_open_overnight/beds_ts08_1.xls;
www.performance.doh.gov.uk/hospitalactivity/data_requests/download/critical_care_beds/ccbed_ts_jul08.xls

Despite these points, designated critical care beds in England make up less than 3% of all inpatient beds (Department of Health Performance Data and Statistics – Beds, 2008) (Figure 1.1). As a result, many patients with potential or actual serious illness are located in general wards; and the numbers of these patients continue to rise. It is difficult to gauge exactly how many patients may be in this category at any one time. In 2002, a snapshot review of 1873 ward patients in four Hospital Trusts found that 12.2% needed care over and above normal ward levels, while a follow-up audit in the same area in 2006 found that 21.3% required such care (Chellel et al, 2002; Smith et al, 2008).

LEARNING OBJECTIVES
By the end of this chapter you should be able to:

❏ Outline reasons for the increased acuity and dependency of patients cared for in general ward areas
❏ Understand/describe the definition of Level 1 care

- ❏ Identify the priorities of rapid assessment and intervention in the acutely ill patient
- ❏ Describe the common framework for assessment of the acutely unwell patient
- ❏ Understand the importance of having/using an effective triggering system to ensure help is called at an appropriate time
- ❏ Understand the importance of communication in ensuring that the patient receives timely and appropriate assistance.

LEVELS OF CARE (INTENSIVE CARE SOCIETY, 2009)

Descriptors of the levels of care needed by different patients have been published by the Intensive Care Society (2009). Level 2 and Level 3 patients will usually be managed in a designated critical care area – if aggressive measures are appropriate. However, as has been noted above, there are many Level 1 patients on wards: these are patients at risk of deterioration or patients recently transferred from a higher level of care whose needs can be met on an acute ward as long as there is additional advice and support from the critical care team (Intensive Care Society, 2009). In this context, it is imperative that staff working in wards are able to recognise (and intervene effectively) when patients deteriorate.

Box 1.1 Level 1 patients

- Patients recently discharged from a higher level of care: e.g. needing at least 4-hourly vital sign observations.
- Patients in need of additional monitoring/clinical interventions, clinical input or advice: e.g. needing at least 4-hourly observations, or continuous oxygen therapy, or boluses of intravenous fluid, or epidural analgesia; or with a tracheostomy or chest drain in situ, or receiving an intravenous infusion of insulin; or needing physiotherapy to prevent or treat respiratory failure.
- Patients requiring critical care outreach service support: e.g. with abnormal vital signs but not (yet) needing a higher level of care; and those at risk of deterioration with a potential requirement for a higher level of care.

ARE WARD STAFF READY FOR THE CHALLENGE?

Nursing staff are the constant monitors of patients' well-being. Nurses must ensure that their knowledge of the patient is not restricted to arm's-length evaluation of data but is based on regular accurate assessments and a good understanding of the patient's physical and mental state. In order to do this, nurses must have an appreciation of what is normal and what is not.

However, at the same time as the acute hospital patient population has changed – and generally become more challenging – there have also been a number of changes to the way that medical and nursing staff are trained and work. These developments have not helped staff to easily become competent in recognising and responding to sudden acute deterioration in patients.

Limited experience with sick patients for medical and nursing staff

Changes in the way that nurses are trained have led to a reduction in time spent gaining 'hands-on' experience with patients. The typical 3-year training for a nursing diploma or degree complies with the Nursing and Midwifery Council requirement for 50% theory and 50% practice (NMC, 2004). It is likely to include a maximum of 2300 hours of total practice experience – or 102 days per year (NMC, 2004) – which must cover all aspects of nursing, thus allowing only a limited time specifically with sick patients.

These changes mean that intuitive recognition of acute deterioration is likely to be less well-developed and will require teaching that is specific to subjective indicators (such as skin colour and behavioural changes) as well as better understanding of the more objective indicators (such as respiratory rate and blood pressure). Ruth-Sahd and Hendy (2005) found that novice nurses depended heavily on intuition and were unable to explain the reasoning behind their decisions. They were more likely to be correct if they were older and had a broad spectrum of social and personal experience. In a study of nurses who had called the emergency team because they were worried, Cioffi (2000) found that in the process of recognition, nurses relied heavily on past experiences and knowledge to detect differences in the patient's condition.

Similar issues have arisen within the medical profession with concerns about the amount of clinical experience of trainee doctors and the impact of foundation year programmes and post-graduate training structures that result in far less time getting 'hands-on' exposure to patients (McManus et al 1998). Senior doctors are also likely to be less experienced than they used to be: a *British Medical Journal* editorial pointed out that it is now possible to become a consultant surgeon with 6000 hours of specialist experience, whereas previously a trainee might expect to work 30,000 hours (Chikwe et al, 2004).

Such deficits need to be addressed by focused teaching that develops and enhances the knowledge and skills required for the recognition and management of acutely ill patients. These include skills of assessment, problem and risk identification and knowledge of appropriate interventions.

PROBLEMS IN ACUTE CARE

Reports from around the world show major healthcare systems struggling to meet the challenge of providing consistently safe and effective care of acutely and critically ill patients (e.g. Australia – Wilson et al, 1995; USA – Kohn et al, 2000). In the United Kingdom, McQuillan et al (1998) examined the care of patients that had deteriorated to the point that they required transfer to intensive care. In a total of 100 patients from two hospitals, only 20 patients were judged to have been well managed, while 54 experienced sub-optimal care in the period before transfer. Outcomes were poor even among those patients considered well-managed, with a mortality rate of 35%; however, in the sub-optimal care group, the mortality rate was 56%. Importantly, the baseline characteristics of the two groups of patients were not significantly different and the difference in mortality can be attributed to the difference in quality of care rather than to differences between the patients themselves. Other studies have also shown the impact of sub-optimal ward care in prestigious teaching hospitals (McGloin et al, 1999; Vincent et al, 2001) and district general hospitals alike (Seward et al, 2003).

As recently as 2005, the National Confidential Enquiry into Patient Outcome and Death (NCEPOD) report of care in 1154 acute medical patients in 179 English hospitals found:

- Initial assessment was unacceptable in 10% of cases
- Initial treatment was delayed and inappropriate in 48% of cases
- Care was less than good practice in 47% of patients, and contributed to death in one-third of the cases.

It is important to emphasise that these problems are often the product of ineffective systems rather than individual lack of skill, knowledge or judgement. McQuillan et al (1998) found that failures of organisation and lack of supervision were significant factors, but also that failure to appreciate clinical urgency and seek advice played a part. Most often, poor patient outcomes are linked to delayed recognition and ineffective management of fundamental aspects of care, such as:

- Ensuring a clear airway
- Optimising breathing and giving oxygen
- Treatment of circulatory failure.
                        (McQuillan et al, 1998; McGloin et al, 1999)

Healthcare workers have an individual and collective responsibility to reflect on their own performance and address any deficits in knowledge or skills as well as to evaluate the strengths and weaknesses of the system as a whole. This approach can form the basis of a high-quality service that works to minimise variability and risk in patient care.

PRIORITIES OF ASSESSMENT AND INTERVENTION
It is essential that all staff are familiar with the clinical priorities in life-threatening situations in order to ensure that problems are identified and treated in the right order. The right order is one that identifies and treats problems that will harm or even kill the patient most rapidly. There is a very clear hierarchy for this.

Key Point

Identify and respond first to what will kill the patient first.

In all cases, problems causing hypoxia and hypotension are potentially life-threatening and should be identified and treated immediately. It is therefore not surprising that the A (Airway), B (Breathing), C (Circulation) format taught on basic and advanced life support courses (Resuscitation Council UK, 2006) and similar programmes equally applies to management of patients that are acutely unwell. Once these priorities have been addressed, other important assessments can be made.

Box 1.2 Definitions

Hypoxia = inadequate availability of oxygen for cell metabolism
Hypotension = low blood pressure
(systolic BP <90 mmHg or decreased by >40 mmHg from normal)

Clearly, if the patient is not seen to be breathing through a clear airway, and/or there is no palpable pulse, a cardiac arrest call should be made and life support commenced.

Key Point

Unresponsive patient or patient with grossly abnormal (or no) breathing or no palpable pulse = Cardiac Arrest Call.

In an acute situation, assessment will initially focus on the patient himself, with most information obtained from a direct examination. However, once any life-threatening problems have been identified or excluded, a more thorough assessment can be made using information from other sources.

Additional sources of information include

- Observation charts
- Fluid balance charts
- Prescription charts
- Blood chemistry/haematology results

- Microbiology results
- Relevant x-rays and scans
- The patient's medical team
- Other healthcare professionals
- The patient's family.

USING AN ASSESSMENT FRAMEWORK FOR INITIAL ASSESSMENT

In an acute situation, it is important to have a simple structure to ensure that priorities are addressed and then that all other relevant issues are considered. A systematic approach should be used; it should highlight the life-threatening problems that must be recognised and responded to first. Most training programmes designed to improve capability in managing the sick patient use the A–B–C–D–E structure (see Table 1.1).

> **Key Point**
>
> Use a systematic approach when assessing a sick patient: this supports identification of the main priorities and ensures that the most important issues are assessed and addressed.

Table 1.1 A systematic framework for priority-driven initial assessment of the sick patient

Category	Assessment	Examples of assessment
A	Airway	Patient is talking Stridor heard
B	Breathing	Chest movement is equal Respiratory rate
C	Circulation	Pulse rate Peripheral temperature or capillary refill
D	Disability	Level of consciousness Pain
E	Examination or Exposure	Obvious inflammation Bleeding

The chapters that follow will expand and explain each step of the assessment framework.

CALLING FOR APPROPRIATE ASSISTANCE

According to local arrangements, each organisation should ensure that there are clear guidelines for calling for help from the patient's own medical team and a Critical Care Outreach service (where this exists). Such guidelines enable the patient to receive an appropriate level of timely, expert support: early interventions can minimise further deterioration and improve outcomes (Newby et al, 1996; Rivers et al, 2001). Conversely, delays in transfer to a critical care unit with the right staff, equipment and expertise are associated with worse outcomes (Parkhe et al, 2002; Young et al, 2003). Outcomes are likely to be worse than they need be should prescribed protocols for managing acutely ill patients not be followed: such cases are clinical governance issues that will require investigation.

Calling for assistance has been shown to be most effective when the correct information and language is used when referring a patient to medical staff. Although nurses tend to use descriptive language among themselves, such as 'Mr Jones has gone off today' or 'I'm worried about Mrs Tate, she isn't herself', this tends to be less effective when requesting a medical review.

Andrews and Waterman (2005) found that use of an early warning score empowered nurses to better communicate physiological deterioration and resulted in a more convincing referral. An effective referral can make the difference between achieving timely treatment rather than a worse outcome for the patient.

Guidelines to calling for help for the acutely ill patient

Cardiac arrest is easily identifiable and summoning assistance from the cardiac arrest team is a clearly prescribed response. However, in other circumstances it may be more difficult to decide when to call for help and how to define the urgency of the call. The Department of Health report *Comprehensive Critical Care* (2000) suggested that Critical Care Outreach services can be used to ensure that patients receive the right level of expert care wherever they are located.

Many hospitals have developed methods, known as Track and Trigger systems, to alert staff to patients that are acutely deteriorating. These systems use physiological signs as call criteria or to give an early warning score that will trigger a response either from an outreach team or from the patient's own medical team (or, ideally, both). These will be explained in more detail in Chapter 2.

CONCLUSION

Overall, there is a need to ensure that there is early recognition of acute deterioration by professionals trained in clinical assessment, interpretation of abnormal physiology and the recognition of critical illness who can then ensure that the patient receives the right treatment at the time that it is needed. These skills are essential for proper patient care and will be explained in the following chapters. Several chapters include clinical scenarios to support application of the skills described to real-life situations.

CHAPTER SUMMARY

Although most people seen in hospital are still unlikely to become seriously ill during their stay, a significant and increasing number of ward patients may experience acute deterioration that requires an increased level of care.

Trends in healthcare such as the shift towards primary care and increased levels of day surgery have resulted in a situation where the acuity and dependency of those patients that are admitted to hospital are rising. Nurses need to monitor such patients and recognise when acute deterioration takes place.

The priorities for assessment and intervention are those factors that will kill the patient most rapidly – i.e. hypoxia and hypotension.

Rapid assessment and intervention should follow a common assessment framework that ensures that Airway, Breathing and Circulation are prioritised but also that other important factors, such as neurological deterioration, or serious problems, such as deep vein thrombosis, are not missed.

Use of a Track and Trigger system with call criteria or an early warning score can ensure that expert help is summoned in a timely manner from medical staff or a Critical Care Outreach team as appropriate.

REFERENCES

Andrews T, Waterman H (2005) Packaging: a grounded theory of how to report physiological deterioration effectively. Journal of Advanced Nursing 52:473–481

Chellel A, Fraser J, Fender V, et al (2002) Nursing observations on ward patients at risk of critical illness. Nursing Times 98:36–39

Chikwe J, de Souza AC, Pepper JR (2004) No time to train the surgeons. British Medical Journal 328:418–419

Cioffi J (2000) Recognition of patients who require emergency assistance: a descriptive study. Heart & Lung 29:262–268

Department of Health (2000) Comprehensive Critical Care: a review of adult critical care services. Department of Health, London

Department of Health Performance Data and Statistics – Beds (2008) (www.dh.gov.uk/en/Publicationsandstatistics/Statistics/Performancedataandstatistics/index.htm)

Hospital Episode Statistics inpatient data, headline figures, 2006–07 (www.hesonline.nhs.uk)

Intensive Care Society (2009) Levels of critical care for adult patients. Intensive Care Society, London

Kohn LT, Corrigan JM, Donaldson MS (Eds) (2000) To Err is Human: building a safer health system. National Academies Press, Washington DC

McGloin H, Adam SK, Singer M (1999) Unexpected deaths and referrals to intensive care of patients on general wards. Journal of the Royal College of Physicians of London 33:255–259

McManus IC, Richards P, Winder BC (1998) Clinical experience of UK medical students. The Lancet 351:802–803

McQuillan P, Pilkington S, Allan A, et al (1998) Confidential inquiry into quality of care before admission to intensive care. British Medical Journal 316:1853–1858

NCEPOD (2005) An Acute Problem? National Confidential Enquiry into Patient Outcome and Death, London

Newby LK, Rutsch WR, Califf RM, et al (1996) Time from symptom onset to treatment and outcomes after thrombolytic therapy. Journal of the American College of Cardiology 27:1646–1655

NHS Confederation (2006) Why we need fewer hospital beds. The NHS Confederation, London

NMC (2004) Standards of proficiency for pre-registration nursing education. Nursing and Midwifery Council, London

Parkhe M, Myles PS, Leach DS, et al (2002) Outcome of emergency department patients with delayed admission to an intensive care unit. Emergency Medicine 14:50–57

Resuscitation Council UK (2006) Advanced Life Support (5th edn). Resuscitation Council UK, London

Rivers E, Nguyen B, Havstad S, et al (2001) Early goal-directed therapy in the treatment of severe sepsis and septic shock. New England Journal of Medicine 345:1368–1377

Ruth-Sahd LA, Hendy HM (2005) Predictors of novice nurses' use of intuition to guide patient care decisions. Journal of Nursing Education 44:450–458

Seward E, Greig E, Preston S, et al (2003) A confidential study of deaths after emergency medical admission: issues relating to quality of care. Clinical Medicine 3:425–434

Smith S, Fraser J, Plowright C, et al (2008) Nursing observations on ward patients – results of a five-year audit. Nursing Times 104:28–29

Vincent C, Neale G, Woloshynowych M (2001) Adverse events in British hospitals: preliminary retrospective record review. British Medical Journal 322:517–519

Wilson RM, Runciman WB, Gibberd RW, et al (1995) The Quality in Australian Healthcare Study. Medical Journal of Australia 163:458–471

Young MP, Gooder VJ, McBride K, et al (2003) Inpatient transfers to the intensive care unit: delays are associated with increased mortality and morbidity. Journal of General Internal Medicine 18:77–83

Track and Trigger Systems: Early Warning Scores, Calling Criteria and Rapid Response Teams

2

INTRODUCTION

The vital importance of systematic assessment to detect physiological deterioration was discussed in Chapter 1: specific observation and assessment techniques are detailed in later chapters. The concepts of early warning scores and calling criteria and the development of rapid response teams have all contributed to the development of track and trigger systems. Patients' physiological signs and symptoms are tracked, and referral to specialist critical care teams is triggered when certain agreed criteria are met. This chapter will discuss the track and trigger concept in more detail and will examine how calling criteria and rapid response teams were created and developed. The physiological calling criteria that make up early warning systems will be examined, and issues with implementation of these systems will be discussed.

LEARNING OBJECTIVES

By the end of this chapter you should be able to:

❑ Discuss the problems of sub-optimal care
❑ Discuss the background to rapid response teams
❑ Identify the main vital signs that help to detect physiological deterioration
❑ Understand how track and trigger systems work
❑ Discuss current national UK policy regarding track and trigger systems

❏ Understand the role that the ward nurse plays in detecting and managing the deteriorating patient.

THE ORIGIN AND DEVELOPMENT OF THE RAPID RESPONSE TEAM CONCEPT

Patients in hospital can experience unexpected physiological deterioration that can lead to critical illness, intensive care unit (ICU) admission, cardiac arrest or death. Much of this deterioration can be signalled in patients' physiological signs, such as pulse, blood pressure and respiratory rate, which can be readily monitored by ward nurses as part of routine practice. However, several American studies in the 1990s found that abnormal physiological signs and symptoms (antecedents) were present in a large number of patients who went on to suffer a cardiac arrest; and it was found that many of these antecedents had been missed, neglected or poorly managed (Schein et al, 1990; Bedell et al, 1991; Franklin and Mathew, 1994; Rich, 1999).

At around the time that American researchers were studying the physiological antecedents to cardiac arrest, there were increasing concerns regarding sub-optimal ward care in Australia. The Medical Emergency Team (MET) concept was developed in a Sydney hospital in 1990 (Lee et al, 1995). The MET was modelled on the principles of rapid detection and correction of vital sign abnormalities previously developed in trauma care. This approach was based on minimising deficiencies in routine clinical management by involving experienced medical staff with appropriate skills as early as possible in the treatment of deteriorating patients (Deane et al, 1989). The purpose of the MET was to rapidly assess and treat seriously ill hospital patients at risk of cardio-pulmonary arrest and other life-threatening events before irreversible deteriorations occurred (Lee et al, 1995). The MET, an experienced critical care team, was alerted by ward staff when the patient showed predetermined abnormal signs.

The influences of the Australian MET concept, along with increasing UK concerns about ward care raised by McQuillan et al (1998), McGloin et al (1999) and Hodgetts et al (2002), resulted in similar pre-emptive teams being developed in the UK (Goldhill et al, 1999). Abnormal physiological criteria were identified to help ward staff detect deteriorating patients and prompt a referral. Goldhill et al (1999) developed the patient-at-risk team (PART) using a multi-parameter system to trigger referral. The criteria chosen to prompt referral to the team were based on face validity, decided by an expert multidisciplinary group at the hospital. The PART system differed from the Australian MET system in that it relied on a number of criteria being met before the PART was called.

Morgan et al (1997) also developed early warning criteria, but without the accompanying team. These criteria were based on a system of scores being attributed to physiological ranges of patient observations, which were added together to result in an aggregated score (Morgan et al, 1997). The criteria were based on observations of patients admitted to ICU, but there were no reports of whether the criteria were tested for specificity or sensitivity. A summary of all three early warning scoring systems can be found in Table 2.1.

Although American researchers had led with studies into the physiological antecedents to cardiac arrest, there is little published evidence that the Americans adopted the early warning systems established in Australia and embraced by the UK. The earliest report of a MET system in the USA was that described by DeVita et al (2004) in a Pittsburgh tertiary care hospital. However, wide-scale adoption of the early warning system concept in America followed in 2005–2006 when the "Saving 100,000 Lives Campaign" was launched by the Institute for Healthcare Improvement (IHI) in 2004 (Institute for Healthcare Improvement, 2005). The Saving Lives Campaign targeted six changes that would make a positive impact on patient outcomes, the first of which was the introduction of Rapid Response Teams. At the end of 2005, the IHI reported that more than 3000 American hospitals (about 80%) had joined the campaign (www.ihi.org).

DEVELOPING EARLY WARNING SCORING (EWS) SYSTEMS AND CRITICAL CARE OUTREACH (CCO) SERVICES IN THE UK

Growing concerns about sub-optimal ward care in the UK were reflected in a report on critical care published by the Audit Commission in 1999, which stated that:

Table 2.1 Summary of the three main early warning systems

	Lee et al (1995)	Goldhill et al (1999)	Morgan et al (1997)
Type of system	Single parameter	Multiple parameter	Aggregated. Five physiological parameters are weighted from a score of 0 (most normal) to 3 (most abnormal)
Condition for calling	Any one criteria	The senior ward nurse should contact the responsible doctor and inform them of a patient with *any three or more* of the referral criteria below	Aggregated score of ≥3
Rationale for criteria	Not specified	Agreed by multidisciplinary expert team in authors' hospital	Locally decided based on analysis of ICU patients
Physiological ranges agreed for referral			
Temperature (°C)	<35.5 or >39.5	Not included	0 = 36.6–37.4 1 = 35.1–36.5 or >37.5 2 = <35
Systolic blood pressure (mmHG)	<100 or >200	<90	0 = 101–199 1 = 81–100 2 = 71–80 or >200 3 = <70
Respiratory rate (breaths/min)	<10 or >30	<10 or ≥25	0 = 9–14 1 = 15–20 2 = <8 or 21–29 3 = >30
Heart rate (beats/min)	<40 or >120	<55 or >110	0 = 51–100 1 = 41–50 or 101–110 2 = <40 or 111 = 130 3 = 130
Urine output	<500 ml in 24 h	<100 ml over previous 4 h	Not included.

Level of consciousness	Decreased or altered	Not fully alert and orientated	0 = Alert 1 = Responds to voice 2 = Responds to pain 3 = Unresponsive Not included
Oxygen saturation	Not included	<90%	Not included
Potassium	<3 or >6		
Sodium	<125 or >155		
Blood sugar	<2 or >20		
Arterial pH	<7.2 or >7.55		
Base Excess	<−15 or >+10		
Other conditions/ situations	New arrhythmia Pulm. oedema Acute severe asthma Acute resp. failure Upper airways obstruction Hypovolaemic, cardiac, anaphylactic or septic shock Acute diabetic emergencies Near drowning Carbon monoxide poisoning Severe drug overdose Amniotic fluid embolism Pre eclampsia Status epilepticus Acute psychiatric disturbance Excessive bleeding Excessive drainage	OR a patient not *fully* alert and orientated AND respiratory rate ≥35 breaths/min OR heart rate ≥140 beats/min. Unless immediate management improves the patient, the doctor should consider calling the team. Exceptionally (in emergency when the responsible doctor is not immediately available), the senior ward nurse may contact the team directly. A doctor of registrar grade or above may call the team for any seriously ill patient causing acute concern. This will normally be done after discussion with the patient's consultant. The consultant responsible for the patient must be informed that the team has been called.	None specified

Critical care units may become the backstop for a poorly performing hospital. Poor general care can result in patients needing critical care. This inflates the number of critical care beds required. Poor care may happen in A&E, the admissions unit, the operating theatre or on the wards. It can happen due to organisational failures, communication breakdowns, failure to seek consultant or specialist advice, failure to spot or act on danger signs, and failures in supervision and on-call response.

(Audit Commission, 1999:48)

Several recommendations came out of the report with the aim of improving the skills of ward nurses and doctors in the detection of critical illness; to agree "danger signs" of deterioration; and to develop outreach services to support ward staff in managing at-risk patients (Audit Commission, 1999).

In 2000, the Department of Health published a review of adult critical care services (Department of Health, 2000). It supported the Audit Commission's (1999) recommendations about the implementation of Critical Care Outreach (CCO) teams and Early Warning Scoring (EWS) systems across England and Wales. Both the EWS and CCO initiatives were intended to avert admissions to the ICU, enable discharges from the ICU, and enhance the critical care skills of ward staff (Department of Health, 2000).

Since the publication of the UK government recommendations (Department of Health, 2000), a variety of models of CCO and EWS have been developed across the country (Department of Health, 2003). The most common CCO team model consists of expert critical care nurses responding to referrals from the wards and working with ward staff in the detection and management of deteriorating patients. The most frequently used model of EWS systems are based on the Morgan et al (1997) model (Department of Health, 2003), but the physiological parameters used, and their weighted ranges, may vary where they have been locally implemented.

In June 2005 a worldwide consensus conference on medical emergency teams was held in Pittsburgh, USA (DeVita et al 2006). Experts in patient safety, hospital and critical care medicine described a Rapid Response System (RRS) that consists of an afferent limb, which included event detection and trigger, and an efferent limb, which consisted of the medical response. The afferent limb involves the bedside nurse monitoring the patient to detect when a patient is at risk or has actual physiological deterioration. Routine observation of temperature, pulse, blood pressure, respiratory rate and oxygen saturation and the use of early warning systems guides the nurse as to when to trigger the expert team. The efferent limb involves the medical response and can be a full medical team, such as the medical emergency team, or a nurse-led service, such as the critical care outreach team.

PHYSIOLOGICAL CALLING CRITERIA

The original early warning scores and calling criteria were developed using expert knowledge and face validity to determine which components of the patient's signs and symptoms – and which values – would be useful in identifying deterioration. The aim of any early warning system is to optimise sensitivity and specificity, while making it as simple as possible for nurses, doctors and other staff to use. The sensitivity of an early warning system is how good it is as detecting deteriorating patients, while the specificity is how good it is at rejecting patients that are not deteriorating. A balance has to be struck between the sensitivity and specificity of an early warning scoring system, and the complexity of the instrument. A system that has too many items to measure, takes too long or needs high levels of skill will not be readily applied in practice.

As track and trigger systems are developing, more evidence is emerging that informs us of the most useful indicators for detecting physiological deterioration. There is a patho-physiological course of deterioration common to most patients with a range of underlying clinical conditions (Smith, 2003), and certain signs can usually be observed as the body responds to reducing organ perfusion. These signs and symptoms will be discussed using the A–B–C–D–E approach, which is part of the systematic process used to structure patient assessment.

AIRWAY AND BREATHING

The initial response of the body to poor organ perfusion is to increase the intake of oxygen, which will be marked by an increase in respiratory rate (RR). Changes in respiratory function have been recognised as one of the most important early signs of deterioration (Schein et al, 1990; Goldhill et al, 1999; Goldhill and McNarry, 2004). Abnormal RR was reported to be associated with risk of cardiac arrest by Hodgetts et al (2002), and high RR was the second most common antecedent to death in another study by Hillman et al (2001). In the ACADEMIA study (Kause et al, 2004), threatened airway and low RR (<5 breaths/min) were the third and fourth most frequent antecedents to cardiac arrest, death and unplanned admission to intensive care. Cuthbertson et al (2007) found that oxygen saturation <96% was a significant predictor of deterioration in surgical high dependency patients, and oxygen saturation levels of 90–95% as well as <90% were also found to be significantly associated with death by Jacques et al (2006). Both RR and oxygen saturation are easy to measure and can be valuable indicators of deterioration. RR parameters are found in all track and trigger systems but oxygen saturation, although common, is not a universal element.

Key Point

Changes in respiratory rate are one of the most important signs of deterioration.

CIRCULATION

The second and third most universal parameter measured in track and trigger systems are heart rate (HR) and systolic blood pressure (SBP). As with RR, increase in HR is an early compensatory mechanism to optimise organ perfusion. Other physiological compensatory mechanisms that occur, such as reduced peripheral perfusion (cool and clammy hands and feet) and reduction in urine output, are all aimed at preserving body fluid in the attempt to maintain adequate blood pressure. So while increase in HR may be an early sign of deterioration, hypotension indicates that the body has decompensated and is a relatively late sign. Abnormal heart rate (<59 and >99 beats/min) has been reported as an important antecedent variable prior to death by Goldhill and McNarry (2004) and the most frequent abnormality prior to intensive care unit admission (Goldhill et al, 1999). Cuthbertson et al (2007) reported that HR >90 beats/min was a significant determinant to predict deterioration in surgical high-dependency patients, and, although Cuthbertson et al (2007) found that SBP was not as good a discriminator to predict deterioration, Hillman et al (2001) found that the commonest physiological abnormality prior to death was hypotension (SBP <90 mmHg), and the second was tachyopneoa (RR >36 breaths/min).

Urine output measurement is also an indication of circulatory efficiency, but is not a common feature in all track and trigger systems. This may be due to the fact that only a relatively small number of patients in hospital have their urine output measured. However, there is evidence that poor urine output (<200 ml per 24 h) has been significantly associated with death (Jacques et al, 2006), and it may be prudent to measure urine output in the deteriorating ward patient.

Core temperature features in a number of track and trigger systems and while it is an important component in the Surviving Sepsis algorithm (Silva et al, 2006), its contribution to predicting physiological deterioration is not proven. Cuthbertson et al (2007) found that temperature was not a good discriminator of deterioration and Goldhill et al (2005) reported that temperature was not associated with hospital mortality.

Other common and simple measures to assess circulation are limb temperature, which has been mentioned above, and capillary refill time. These tend not to be featured in track and trigger systems but are important assessment techniques and they are discussed more fully in later chapters.

Key Point

If the patient is deteriorating it may be useful to measure urine output for a 24-hour period to ensure adequate kidney perfusion.

DISABILITY (MENTAL STATE)

Adequate cerebral perfusion is very sensitive to changes in mean arterial pressure, and hypoxic and poorly perfused patients will often show signs of mental impairment, including new irritability, agitation, confusion and low levels of consciousness. Therefore, assessing the patient's mental state will give early indications of deterioration.

Disability is commonly assessed by evaluating the patient's conscious level and a simple measure used in track and trigger systems is the AVPU assessment: Is the patient Alert? Is the patient responding to your Voice? Does the patient respond to Pain? Or, is the patient Unresponsive? More advanced assessment incorporates the Glasgow Coma Scale (GCS). Both assessment tools will be discussed more fully in a later chapter.

Low levels of consciousness feature as a significant antecedent to an adverse event in patients in a number of studies. Schein et al (1990) reported that changes in mental state were a feature in 27 out of 64 patients (42%) who went on to have a cardiac arrest. Jacques et al (2006) also found that changes in mentation were associated with cardiac arrest and death and Hodgetts et al (2002) reported that a low GCS was a significant feature prior to cardiac arrest.

By combining the elements of the early warning score that may be implemented in your organisation, and the observation and assessment of other physical signs of the patient using the A–B–C–D–E approach, it is possible to produce a comprehensive appraisal of the patient's condition. Ongoing assessment will give information about whether the patient's condition is improving or deteriorating, as well as the response to any treatments.

Key Point

Reduced consciousness can cause airway obstruction and death, and should be considered a medical emergency.

THE ROLE OF THE NURSE IN VITAL SIGNS MONITORING, EWS AND CCO

It has long been accepted that it is the nurses' role to take and record patients' vital signs while in hospital. Florence Nightingale stated that:

The most important practical lesson that can be given to nurses is to teach them 1. what to observe; 2. how to observe; 3. what symptoms indicate improvement; 4. what the reverse; ...(Nightingale, 1860, p. 119)

However, undertaking patient observations has been viewed as one of the more mundane tasks of the nurse (Kenward et al, 2001) and has more recently often been delegated to the Health Care Assistant. Traditionally the vital signs have consisted of temperature (T), heart rate (HR), respiratory rate (RR) and blood pressure (BP) (Evans et al, 2001), but newer, additional measures such as pulse oximetry (SpO_2) have been considered useful too (Lockwood et al, 2004).

With the development of early warning systems, the monitoring and recording of vital signs observations has been highlighted as an essential first link in the chain of early recognition of patient deterioration. However, even when EWS systems are in place, and ward staff have access to expert critical care teams, failure to undertake sufficient vital sign monitoring or failure to adhere to EWS protocols continues to be a problem on general hospital wards. In Australia, where the MET system is more advanced, studies have shown that in spite of ready access to METs, nurses on the ward remain reluctant to summon them (Crispin and Daffurn, 1998; Cioffi, 2000). More recently, a large cluster-randomised controlled trial involving 23 hospitals in Australia reported a lack of recorded observations of patients, and lack of referral to MET even when calling criteria were present in patients (Hillman et al, 2005). In the UK, a study conducted by the National Confidential Enquiry into Patient Outcome and Death (NCEPOD, 2005) reported a similar lack of basic physiological observations, and delayed referral to expert help.

The effectiveness of EWS and subsequent referrals to CCO teams are wholly reliant on nurses on the ward performing timely vital signs observations, having a basic understanding of abnormal physiological signs and calling for expert help when required. The Rapid Response Team (RRT) structure containing the afferent and efferent limbs (DeVita et al, 2006) discussed above is similar to the system advocated by the UK National Institute for Health and Clinical Excellence (NICE) in its 2007 document relating to acutely ill patients in hospital. NICE (2007) described a chain of response to the deteriorating patient that starts with 'event detection' in the form of patient observation. It is recognised that this initial observation of the patient may be undertaken by non-clinical staff, patients themselves or even visitors, as well as by clinical staff. When a change in the patient's condition has been noted, the second step involves the recording of observations and further measurements to gain more information. These observations and measurements are then interpreted to confirm and identify the change in the patients' condition, which prompts adjustments to the frequency and level of monitoring. At this stage, clinical treatment may be needed and more senior help required. If the patient fails to respond to initial treatment measures, a secondary management plan is implemented and again more expert help may be needed. This *chain of response* process is set out in Figure 2.1.

Both the DeVita et al (2006) and the NICE (2007) model illustrate an ideal sequence of events that should take place when the patient deteriorates in hospital. However, we have seen how this system can fail to achieve its intended effect in the detection and management of deteriorating ward patients, with resultant suboptimal care and poor patient outcome. By assessing each stage of the process it is possible to highlight the risks inherent in the process, and to start to clarify what practices may hinder or enhance the process. To this end, using the process mapping from both the DeVita et al (2006) model and the NICE (2007) model, as well as stages in risk assessment, a risk assessment model for the deteriorating ward patient can highlight the six steps in the recognition and management of the deteriorating ward patient and the possible associated risks to the process. The risk assessment model is highlighted in Figure 2.2.

CONCLUSION

The effective detection and management of the deteriorating ward patient is largely reliant on the ward nurses performing timely vital signs observations, having a basic understanding of abnormal physiological signs and calling for expert help when required. Where there are early warning scoring systems and critical care outreach teams in place, their success is dependent

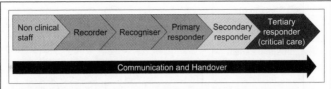

Non-clinical supporter who may also be the 'alerter' and may include the patient or visitor

The recorder who takes designated measurements and records observations and information

The recogniser who monitors the patients' condition, interprets designated measurements, observations and information, and adjusts the frequency of observations and level of monitoring

The primary responder who goes beyond recording and further observation by interpreting the measurements and initiating a clinical management plan: e.g. commencing oxygen therapy; insertion of airway adjuncts; selection of intravenous fluids and administration of a bolus

The secondary responder who is likely to be called to attend when the patient fails to respond to the primary intervention, or continues to 'trigger' or 're-trigger' a response. This individual will assess the clinical effect of the primary intervention, formulate a diagnosis, refine the management plan, initiate a secondary response and will have the knowledge to recognise when referral to critical care is indicated

Tertiary responder. This role will be undertaken by staff possessing appropriate critical care competencies such as advanced airway management, resuscitation, and clinical examination and interpretation of critically ill patients

Fig. 2.1 The chain of response (NICE, 2007)
Reproduced under the terms of the Click-Use Licence

on the ward nurse recording vital signs and complying with referral criteria. There is still much work to be done to define which parameters are the most useful to measure and what their weighted ranges may be. We can also continue to work with ward nurses and doctors to improve their knowledge and skill in physiological assessment techniques. By bringing teams who have specialist knowledge together, we can optimise clinical decision making and improve patient outcomes.

If effective and timely observation of the ward patient is the first step in the successful management of deteriorating ward patients, it is vital we have a better understanding of the physiology of deterioration, and also of how teams work together to

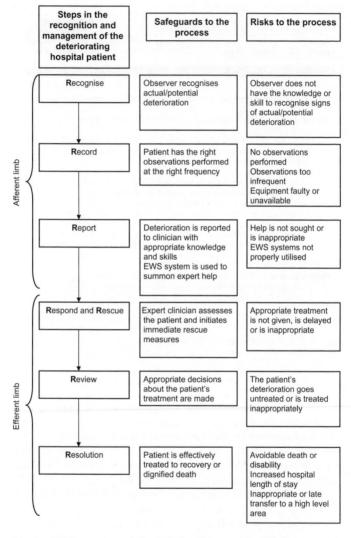

Fig. 2.2 Risk assessment model for the deteriorating ward patient

ensure EWS and CCO have the positive impact on patient outcome that they have the potential to achieve.

CHAPTER SUMMARY

Concerns with the problem of the deteriorating ward patient not being recognised or properly managed has led to the development of rapid response systems using early warning triggers to support ward staff in the care of the acutely ill patient.

These systems have been developed in Australia and America as well as the UK. There are some common physiological signs and symptoms that are utilised in the early warning systems and there are varying levels of evidence to support their utility.

Patient safety is high on the national health agenda in the UK and a number of key reports are a useful resource for understanding this issue.

The bedside nurse plays a vital role in the detection and management of the deteriorating patient and training in patient assessment skills is an important component of the process.

REFERENCES

Audit Commission (1999). Critical to Success. Audit Commission, London

Bedell SE, Deitz DC, Leeman D, Delbanco, TL (1991) Incidence and characteristics of preventable iatrogenic cardiac arrests. Journal of the American Medical Association 266(21):2815–2820

Cioffi J (2000) Nurses' experience of making decisions to call emergency assistance to their patients. Journal of Advanced Nursing 32(1):108–114

Crispin C, Daffurn K (1998) Nurses' responses to acute severe illness. Australian Critical Care 11(4): 131–133

Cuthbertson BH, Boroujerdi M, et al (2007) Can physiological variables and early warning scoring systems allow early recognition of the deteriorating surgical patient? Critical Care Medicine 35(2):402–409

Deane SA, Gaudry PL, et al (1989) Implementation of a trauma team. Australian and New Zealand Journal of Surgery 59(5):373–378

Department of Health (2000) Comprehensive Critical Care: A review of adult critical care services. Department of Health. The Stationery Office, London

Department of Health (2003) The National Outreach Report. The NHS Modernisation Agency, Department of Health, London

DeVita M, Braithwaite R, et al (2004) Use of medical emergency team responses to reduce hospital cardiopulmonary arrests. Quality Safety in Health Care 13(4):251–254

DeVita MA, Bellomo R, et al (2006) Findings of the first consensus conference on medical emergency teams. Critical Care Medicine 34(9):2463–2478

Evans D, Hodgkinson B, et al (2001) Vital signs in hospital patients: A systematic review. International Journal of Nursing Studies 38(6):643–650

Franklin C, Mathew J (1994) Developing strategies to prevent in-hospital cardiac arrest: Analysing responses of physicians and nurses in the hours before the event. Critical Care Medicine 22(2):244–247

Goldhill DR, White SA, et al (1999) Physiological values and procedures in the 24h before ICU admission from the ward. Anaesthesia 54:529–534

Goldhill DR, McNarry AF et al (2005) A physiologically-based early warning score for ward patients: the association between score and outcome. Anaesthesia 60(6):547–553

Hillman KM, Bristow PJ, et al (2001) Antecedents to hospital deaths. Internal Medicine Journal 31:343–348

Hillman KM, Chen J, et al (2005) Introduction of the medical emergency team (MET) system: A cluster-randomised controlled trial. The Lancet 365(9477):2091–2097

Hodgetts TJ, Kenward G, et al (2002). Incidence, location and reasons for avoidable in-hospital cardiac arrest in a district general hospital. Resuscitation 54(2):115–123

Institute for Healthcare Improvement (2005). www.ihi.org.

Jacques T, Harrison GA, et al (2006) Signs of critical conditions and emergency responses (SOCCER): A model for predicting adverse events in the inpatient setting. Resuscitation 69(2):175–183

Kause J, Smith G, et al (2004) A comparison of antecedents to cardiac arrests, deaths and emergency intensive care admissions in Australia and New Zealand, and the United Kingdom – the ACADEMIA study. Resuscitation 62:275–282

Kenward G, Hodgetts TJ, et al (2001) Time to put the R back in TPR. Nursing Times 97(40):32–33

Lee A, Bishop G, et al (1995) The Medical Emergency Team. Anaesthesia and Intensive Care 23(2):183–186

Lockwood C, Conroy-Hiller T, Page T (2004) Vital Signs. Joanna Briggs Institute 2:207–230

McGloin H, Adam SK, et al (1999) Unexpected deaths and referrals to intensive care of patients on general wards. Are some cases potentially avoidable? Journal of the Royal College of Physicians of London 33(3): 255–259

McQuillan P, Pilkington S, et al (1998) Confidential inquiry into quality of care before admission to intensive care. British Medical Journal 316(7148):1853–1858

Morgan RJM, Williams F, et al (1997) An early warning system for detecting developing critical illness. Clinical Intensive Care 8(2):100

NICE (2007) Acutely Ill Patients in Hospital. National Institute for Health and Clinical Excellence, London

NCEPOD (2005) An Acute Problem? National Confidential Enquiry into Patient Outcome and Death, London

Nightingale F (1860) Notes on Nursing. Tempus Publishing, Stroud

Rich K (1999) Inhospital cardiac arrest: Pre-event variables and nursing response. Clinical Nurse Specialist 13(3):147–153; quiz 154–156

Schein RMH, Hazday N, et al (1990) Clinical antecedents to in-hospital cardiopulmonary arrest. Chest 98(6):1338–1392

Silva E, Akamine N, et al (2006) Surviving sepsis campaign: A project to change sepsis trajectory. Endocrine Metabolic and Immune Disorders Drug Targets 6(2):217–222

Smith G (2003) ALERT. Acute Life Threatening Events Recognition and Treatment. University of Portsmouth

3 | Assessment Techniques

INTRODUCTION

Nurses have commonly focused on the measurement of observations as their main method of assessing patients. However, to fully understand acute deterioration there are other assessment skills that are required; and it is important that nurses are competent in the application of these skills in acute situations. The best way to achieve competency is to practise such skills as part of clinical simulations or to ensure that they are used during routine assessments of well patients.

LEARNING OBJECTIVES

By the end of this chapter you should be able to

❏ Describe and define the four key components of physical assessment
❏ Identify the key advantages to each component of assessment
❏ Describe the abnormal signs that can be obtained from inspection
❏ Describe auscultation and the technique for using a stethoscope correctly
❏ Describe the abnormal signs from auscultation
❏ Describe the information available from palpation
❏ Describe the abnormal signs from palpation
❏ Understand the contribution of subjective indicators of deterioration to assessment
❏ List other sources of information

The four key components of physical assessment are inspection, palpation, auscultation and percussion. These are defined in Table 3.1.

Table 3.1 Definition of assessment techniques

Assessment technique	Definition
Inspection	Use of visual skills to gather information on a particular system, or the patient as a whole. Utilises both the naked eye and various instruments including ophthalmoscope, auroscope, specula and additional lighting sources
Palpation	Application of the sense of touch to assess texture, temperature, moisture, organ location and size, swelling, vibration, pulsation, rigidity/spasticity, crepitation, masses and pain
Percussion	Tapping of the skin with short, sharp strokes to assess underlying structures. Characteristic sound depicts the location, size and density of underlying organs. It also encompasses use of a 'percussion hammer' to elicit deep tendon reflexes
Auscultation	Listening to sounds produced by the body, such as the heart, blood vessels, lungs and abdomen using a stethoscope

PRIMARY ASSESSMENT

A simple, systematic, priority-driven initial assessment is an essential first step in ensuring an acutely ill patient receives timely and appropriate care. This should follow the A–B–C–D–E priorities discussed in Chapter 1. It can be followed by a more comprehensive secondary assessment once the patient is known to be safe.

All professionals should possess a level of competence fitting with their job roles to undertake patient assessment and to respond to any problem identified. NICE guidance (2007) suggests a 'Chain of Response' should be in place (see Figure 3.1), which aims at being timely, effective, and seamless. Different professional groups may contribute to different parts of the chain according to the local setting. The most important requirement is that the 'overall team' possesses competencies that cover assessment, recognition, intervention and communication to ensure help is obtained when needed (see Chapter 9 for further details).

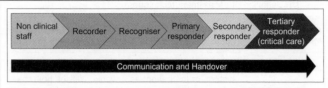

Non-clinical supporter who may also be the 'alerter' and may include the patient or
visitor

The recorder who takes designated measurements and records observations and
information

The recogniser who monitors the patients' condition, interprets designated
measurements, observations and information, and adjusts the frequency of
observations and level of monitoring

The primary responder who goes beyond recording and further observation by
interpreting the measurements and initiating a clinical management plan: e.g.
commencing oxygen therapy; insertion of airway adjuncts; selection of
intravenous fluids and administration of a bolus

The secondary responder who is likely to be called to attend when the patient fails
to respond to the primary intervention, or continues to 'trigger' or 're-trigger'
a response. This individual will assess the clinical effect of the primary
intervention, formulate a diagnosis, refine the management plan, initiate a
secondary response and will have the knowledge to recognise when referral to
critical care is indicated

Tertiary responder. This role will be undertaken by staff possessing appropriate
critical care competencies such as advanced airway management,
resuscitation, and clinical examination and interpretation of critically ill
patients

Fig. 3.1 The chain of response (NICE, 2007)
Reproduced under the terms of the Click-Use Licence

 Look: Visual Assessment or inspection

Throughout the book, this will be referred to as the initial part of
the assessment. This is because a great deal of information can
be picked up from visual inspection and it can continue while
undertaking other parts of the assessment. Most nurses will be
able to pick up on cues that a patient is becoming unwell either
knowingly or unknowingly. These cues include things like

Box 3.1 Techniques

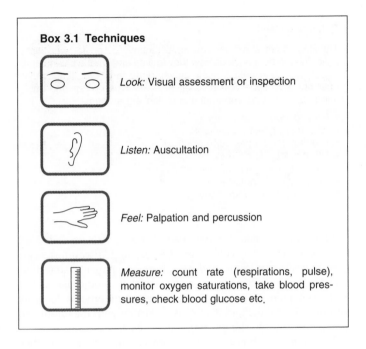

Look: Visual assessment or inspection

Listen: Auscultation

Feel: Palpation and percussion

Measure: count rate (respirations, pulse), monitor oxygen saturations, take blood pressures, check blood glucose etc.

changes in behaviour (e.g. the patient is usually chatty but is now sleepy and unable to maintain a conversation, or the patient was previously willing to try to move around or get out of bed but now lacks energy and is reluctant to move), facial expression (e.g. grimacing or frowning), position (e.g. tensing, hunched over), using accessory muscles to breathe (e.g. rigid neck and shoulder muscles to increase inspiratory capacity). These signs are often seen as the patient is greeted and will allow early recognition of the need for further more detailed assessment.

A global visual assessment can be made with a first approach to the patient (see the Reflective Point below). This will pick up any initial cues. A more detailed inspection should then be made during progression through the A–B–C–D–E system.

Reflective Point

Thinking about a patient you have recently cared for who was critically ill, reflect back on how they looked and what was unusual about their skin colour, their movements, their breathing, their position, the expression on their face, their behaviour and anything else that was apparent just by looking at them.

- *How responsive were they?*
- *Was there chest movement?*
- *Did they have eyes open or shut?*
- *What colour was the skin?*
- *Was there any sign of sweating?*
- *Did they look comfortable?*
- *What position did they adopt?*

Many of the factors mentioned above – such as decreased responsiveness, skin colour, restlessness and discomfort – are sensitive early indicators of deterioration in a patient's condition. Of course, these changes can also be related to other issues like increased pain; it is part of the assessment process to work through potential alternative causes starting with the life-threatening ones and working through the priorities.

If a patient exhibits any of the abnormal signs in Table 3.2 then further assessment is required to understand what is causing them. Signs like these should not be ignored and, although they are very non-specific, they are also likely to be quite significant. In most cases, a full physical assessment and measurement of physiological parameters will be needed.

 Auscultation

Use of a stethoscope to listen to lungs, heart and abdomen can give useful additional information in the acute situation. However, the technique requires practice and exposure to listening to many normal and pathological sounds before it can be used effectively, particularly in emergency situations.

Table 3.2 Visual inspection: normal and abnormal signs

	Normal	Abnormal
Skin colour	Pink/brown Mucosa are pink	Pale, grey/blue tinge Lips and mucosa are purple, pale pink or blue
Responsiveness	Eyes open, or open in response to voice Able to stay awake without constant stimulation	Unresponsive or eyes open only in response to pain Drowsy or falls asleep as soon as any stimulation stops
Facial expression	Relaxed but aware; not frowning, grimacing or tight-lipped	Grimacing, frowning, tight-lipped Slack facial expression and drooling or tongue hanging out
Position	Comfortable in any position	Unable to tolerate specific positions (e.g. unable to lie flat in pulmonary oedema or airway compromise, unable to sit or stand up in hypotension) Rigid shoulder girdle and use of chest/arm splinting to increase chest expansion (e.g. in COPD)
Tension in specific muscles	Relaxed muscle groups at ease in most positions	Tension, guarding over specific painful areas; increased use of accessory muscles of respiration
Behaviour	Gives appropriate answers to questions; able to concentrate for several minutes on specific focus	Appears confused and inappropriate; unable to concentrate on conversation; attempts to get out of bed/walk when unable to do so

Stethoscope technique

The stethoscope consists of a length of tubing which divides into two, ending in soft plastic earpieces. At the other end of the tubing there is a diaphragm on one side and a bell on the other which transmit sound via the tubing and earpieces. The bell is used to hear low-pitched sounds and the diaphragm to hear high-pitched sounds such as normal heart sounds. The diaphragm is recommended for listening to general respiratory sounds (Welsby et al, 2003). The earpieces should be placed snugly in the ears, facing forwards towards the front of the ear. The diaphragm (or bell) of the stethoscope should be placed directly on the patient's skin as listening through clothing can give extraneous sounds that may be difficult to interpret. A systematic sequence of placement should be followed in order to be able to compare both sides of the lungs and to ensure that all lobes are covered (see Chapter 5). The abnormal sounds associated with common respiratory problems are summarised in Table 3.3.

 Palpation

Feeling for areas of tenderness, inflammation, swelling and oedema as well as for the presence of surgical emphysema is part of the general assessment (see Table 3.4). These signs and symptoms tend to be specific to other findings such as underlying infection, haematoma or lymphadenopathy.

Feeling the position of the trachea
Feeling for shift or deviation of the trachea is an important component of respiratory assessment. The trachea should sit directly behind the suprasternal notch. Deviation towards one side or the other suggests either pneumothorax or major pleural effusion (trachea is deviated away from the problem side) or lung collapse (trachea is deviated towards the problem side).

Feeling the pulse
Important information can be obtained from feeling the patient's radial pulse to assess the rate and also regularity and volume.

- Regularity Missed beats can be due to ventricular ectopics. Irregularity can also be caused by atrial fibrillation and other

Table 3.3 Pattern of signs for common respiratory problems

	Consolidation	Pleural effusion	Lobar collapse	Pneumothorax	Pleural thickening
Chest xray					
Mediastinal shift	No	No or away	Towards	No (simple), away (tension)	No
Chest wall excursion	Normal or decreased	Decreased	Decreased	Normal or decreased	Decreased
Percussion note	Normal or decreased	Decreased (stony)	Decreased	Increased	Decreased
Breath sounds	Increased (bronchial)	Decreased	Decreased	Decreased	Decreased
Added sounds	Crackles	Rub (occasional)	None	Click (occasional)	None
Tactile vocal tremitus/ vocal resonance	Increased	Decreased	Decreased	Decreased	Decreased

From Singh S, Rees J (1997) Basics of Respiratory Medicine: 2. Examination. Student BMJ 5(9), with permission from the BMJ Publishing Group

Table 3.4 Physical signs indicating abnormality during palpation

Symptom	Indicator
Tenderness	Patient will report pain or may move to protect the area
Inflammation	The skin will appear reddened and feel warm to touch
Oedema	The skin will appear swollen and tense and will remain indented if pressed
Surgical emphysema	Crackles/popping will be felt under the skin when pressed

abnormal rhythms. If an irregular pulse is felt during assessment, a 12-lead ECG is essential to more fully assess the patient's heart rhythm.

- Volume A high volume (bounding) pulse is associated with sepsis (overwhelming infection). A low volume, difficult to feel pulse is associated with hypotension caused by either hypovolaemia or cardiac dysfunction.

Percussion

This technique is less commonly used but can be useful for detecting levels of fluid, air or organ size in the body cavity. The technique uses both hands, one being laid over the surface to be percussed whilst the middle finger of the other hand strikes with a sharp tap on to the middle finger of the opposite hand. The change in sound indicates differing underlying densities. Tissue and fluid produce a dull sound, air produces a loud or resonant sound and muscle and bone produce a flat sound.

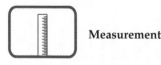 **Measurement**

For measurement of patient observations to be meaningful, the technique must be as accurate as possible. A blood pressure reading that is taken with the wrong size cuff can produce a clinically significant error (>10 mmHg higher or lower) in over 60% of patients (Bur et al, 2000). Similarly, the accuracy of pulse oximetry can be affected by a number of factors, which should be controlled so as to ensure an accurate reading (see Chapter 5).

> **Key Point**
>
> **Ensuring correct BP cuff size**
>
> Bladder width should encircle 40–50% of upper arm circumference.
> Bladder length should cover 80% of the upper arm.
> Cuff and manometer should sit at the level of the heart.

SUBJECTIVE MARKERS OF DETERIORATION USED BY NURSES

It is clear that experienced nurses are capable of detecting very subtle changes in patients as early indicators of acute deterioration (Cioffi, 2000; Andrews and Waterman, 2005). This understanding seems to be dependent on the nurse's experience and level of previous exposure to this type of situation (see Table 3.5), and can be key to the recognition of patient deterioration: therefore these signs should be given the same weight as measured values. Some track and trigger systems recognise this point and 'nurse worried' has been incorporated in a number of systems as a recognised call criterion.

Table 3.5 Subjective indicators of deterioration used by nurses when calling for expert help

Indicator	Process Used	Reference
Feeling 'not right'	Listening, feeling, sensing, knowing	Cioffi (2000)
Colour/clamminess	Observing, touching	Cioffi (2000), Andrews and Waterman (2005)
Agitation	Observing	Cioffi (2000)
Observations marginally changed or not changed at all	Sensing, knowing	Cioffi (2000)

SOURCES OF INFORMATION (OTHER THAN THE PATIENT)

Even in an emergency, valuable information can be found from the patient's charts. If the nurse caring for the patient is involved, most of this data will be known already, but in the situation of a more senior nurse called by a junior or unqualified colleague this information will be needed in order to fully assess the patient.

Blood results

These will add to the picture of what is happening with the patient but a good knowledge of normal limits is required to interpret blood results. Specific relevant blood results will be discussed as part of the assessment in each chapter. As a primary overview, Box 3.2 outlines what should be assessed.

Box 3.2 Primary assessment investigations to be reviewed

Biochemistry	Urea, creatinine and electrolytes (potassium, sodium)
	Blood glucose
	Blood gases: pH, pO_2, pCO_2, standard bicarbonate, base excess/deficit (see Appendix 1)
Haematology	Full blood count: Hb, white cell count, platelets, neutrophils
	Clotting screen
Microbiology	Blood cultures, sputum, urine, CSF
Radiology	Chest x-ray
ECG	12 lead

Patients' notes

Notes are an invaluable source of information, but it can be extremely difficult to sort through and obtain meaningful information from paper notes when you are in a hurry. The nurse at the bedside will be expected to be familiar with the patient history but if the patient has just been admitted or transferred to your care then you may need to access information quickly in situations of acute deterioration.

The most useful source of fast information about current problems and diagnoses is usually a recent full review by a senior member of the patient's medical team. This may constitute part of a transfer letter or may be a recent review in the emergency department or on admission to the ward. If this is unobtainable, physiotherapy reviews are often very thorough.

SUMMARY

Having collected all the information during the assessment, the most important part is still ahead. The information must be sorted, assimilated, analysed and used to make deductions and inferences in order to correctly identify key problems. Even this would be insufficient if the correct responses do not then follow. Thus recognition of a problem such as sepsis resulting from a chest infection causing hypoxaemia and hypotension must be responded to with oxygen, positioning, humidification and physiotherapy as well as communicating with the medical team to ensure nebulisers, antibiotics and intravenous fluids are prescribed as appropriate.

The opportunity to work through and develop this understanding will be given using clinical scenarios in the following chapters.

REFERENCES

Andrews T, Waterman H (2005) Packaging: A grounded theory of how to report physiological deterioration effectively. Journal of Advanced Nursing 52:473–481

Bur A, Hirschl MM, Herkner H, et al (2000) Accuracy of oscillometric blood pressure measurement according to the relation between cuff size and upper-arm circumference in critically ill patients. Critical Care Medicine 28:371–376

Cioffi J (2000) Recognition of patients who require emergency assistance: A descriptive study. Heart & Lung 29:262–268

How to use a stethoscope: www.nursingtimes.net/ntclinical/respiratory_auscultation_how_to_use_a_stethoscope.html

Jarvis C (1996) Physical Examination and Health Assessment (2nd edn). WB Saunders, Philadelphia; cited in Rushforth et al (1998) British Journal of Nursing 7:966–970

NICE (2007) Acutely Ill Patients in Hospital. National Institute for Health and Clinical Excellence, London

Singh S, Rees J (1997) Basics of Respiratory Medicine: 2. Examination. Student BMJ 5(9). www.student.bmj.com/back_issues/0297/data/0297ed1.htm

Welsby PD, Parry G, Smith D (2003) The stethoscope: some preliminary investigations. Postgraduate Medical Journal 79:695–698

A–B–C–D–E: Airway Assessment and Management Techniques

4

INTRODUCTION

The patient's airway is vital – without a clear (patent) airway, the patient will rapidly develop hypoxia, stop breathing and die. Assessing the airway is the most important assessment a nurse can make and is therefore always completed first in any acute situation. Complete airway occlusion will leave the patient only with enough oxygen in their lungs for approximately 3 to 4 minutes. In this short time, circulating oxygen levels will be very low, leading to ischaemia and cell death.

The organs that require the highest levels of oxygen delivery will suffer first. These are the brain, the heart and the kidneys.

LEARNING OBJECTIVES

At the end of this chapter you should be able to:

❑ Recognise complete and partial airway obstruction
❑ Understand the need for speed in assessment and intervention to ensure airway patency
❑ List causes of airway obstruction
❑ Describe methods of maintaining the airway
❑ Outline suction technique for airway/bronchial suction
❑ Identify the point at which expert help is needed (using the clinical scenarios).

ASSESSING THE AIRWAY

Look at the patient as you approach them and, if they are conscious, greet them and ask how they are feeling. This is a very useful high-level assessment. If the patient is able to speak to you, then the airway is patent, and there is sufficient move-

ment of air to allow the vocal cords to be activated. However, speech does not necessarily mean that all is completely well and there may still be some partial airway obstruction. If the patient has partial airway obstruction, their skin colour can be altered to grey, blue or purple, although in the very early stages of choking they may appear very red in the face.

Respiratory effort will be greatly increased and the patient will appear to be making enormous efforts to breathe using accessory muscles such as the neck, pectoral and trapezius muscles for inspiration and the abdominal and internal intercostal muscles for expiration. The patient's breathing maybe paradoxical – i.e. instead of both chest and abdomen moving in the same direction during inspiration or expiration, they will move in opposite directions. So, when the chest lifts and the ribcage moves out-wards, the abdomen will be drawn inwards and vice versa. If the patient is still conscious, then they will be distressed and making desperate attempts to breathe or cough to clear the airway.

Box 4.1 Understanding the need for speed

How long has the patient with an occluded airway got before irreversible hypoxia occurs and the patient dies? The answer is approximately 3–4 minutes.

The lungs contain approximately 5 litres of air, of which oxygen may be only 14% (water vapour in humidified air reduces the ratio of oxygen compared with the atmosphere). This is around 700 ml of oxygen, not all of which can be extracted. The body requires approximately 200 ml of oxygen per minute (this is in a resting state; it will be more if the patient is making huge efforts to breathe). Hence, this gives about 3–4 minutes of oxygen available to the body.

In some cases, where the cause of airway obstruction is also preventing swallowing of saliva, the patient may exhibit constant drooling and again this is an indicator of serious airway obstruction (Box 4.1).

RECOGNISING COMPLETE OR PARTIAL AIRWAY OBSTRUCTION

 Listening to the patient breathing is one of the most useful ways of assessing the airway. It is an important part of the assessment and will provide invaluable information. Although auscultation using a stethoscope will provide the most detailed information, in extreme situations it is often possible to hear symptomatic sounds without a stethoscope.

Complete airway obstruction

If there are no sounds heard from movement of air and no rise and fall of the chest, then the patient has complete airway obstruction. The patient will look grey/blue and will, of course, also be unresponsive.

This is an emergency situation: you should call for help using emergency buzzers or shouting for assistance and immediately attempt to clear the airway (follow UK Resuscitation Council (2006) guidelines for management). The cardiac arrest team should be called. Methods for then managing the airway are discussed later in the chapter.

Partial airway obstruction

This is characterised by altered sounds from air being forced through a restricted passage. Different sounds are caused by different types of obstruction but any of these suggest that the airway is compromised and the patient requires immediate assistance.

- *Snoring* is caused by turbulent air flow through a narrowed upper airway occurring when the soft tissues of the throat, tongue and soft palate are relaxed (as in sleep, low levels of consciousness, coma). These tissues also vibrate during inspiration, contributing to the sound. Snoring may be benign and its significance should be assessed in line with other clinical symptoms such as increased or decreased respiratory rate, ability to respond, and oxygen saturation.

- *Wheezing* is a high-pitched sound caused by air flow through narrowed smaller airways such as bronchioles. It is more commonly heard during expiration but can also occur in inspiration.
- *Stridor* is a harsh, high-pitched sound also caused by turbulent air flow through narrowed airways. This most commonly occurs in inspiration as a result of collapse of the extra-thoracic airways due to increased negative pressure generated by the narrowed airway. It can also occur during expiration. It is a symptom of significant airway obstruction and should not be ignored.
- *Gurgling* is associated with liquid in the airways, which can be mucus, secretions, gastric contents, saliva or any oral intake that has been inhaled. If the patient has a competent cough reflex this will be triggered and the liquid cleared. However, if consciousness level is depressed the patient will have to be assisted to clear this material using oropharyngeal or even tracheal suction.

Other important indicators that the airway may be at risk are less specific but should alert the nurse to potential airway obstruction. These are:

- Hoarse voice: if the patient complains of a hoarse voice which is new and there is no obvious cause (such as recent laryngitis), this may indicate vocal cord dysfunction which can cause airway obstruction.
- Breathing difficulty when lying flat (orthopnoea) or having to sleep sitting upright. This can also be related to pulmonary oedema and cardiac failure as well as airway obstruction. It is a serious sign and the cause should always be investigated.

Reflective Point

Think how you can reassure yourself about the patency of a patient's airway.
What are the best and most immediate ways of assessing this?

CAUSES OF AIRWAY OBSTRUCTION

Obstruction can occur either from blockage inside the airway or from external pressure on the airway causing it to collapse (Boxes 4.2 and 4.3).

One of the most common causes of airway obstruction is the patient's own tongue (Figure 4.1). If the patient is so deeply unconscious that the muscles maintaining the position of the base of the tongue become completely relaxed and the normal reflex mechanisms are blunted, then the patient lying on their back will not be able to prevent the tongue slipping back and covering the airway. This, of course, is the reason that unconscious, deeply sedated or anaesthetised patients should be nursed on their side (in the coma position) unless their airway is being maintained manually (head tilt/chin lift or jaw thrust techniques – Figures 4.2 and 4.3) or with use of an oropharyngeal (guedel) airway (Figure 4.4).

INITIAL MANAGEMENT OF AIRWAY OBSTRUCTION

Immediate establishment of an open airway is vital. This can be done initially by manual head and neck positioning, use of suction or if there is real likelihood of a foreign body, then use of

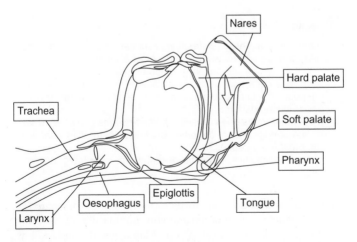

Fig. 4.1 Blocking of airway by base of tongue

Box 4.2 Causes of internal upper airway obstruction

- Vomit
- Secretions
- Blood
- Foreign bodies (e.g. peanut, coin etc.)
- Gastric fluid
- Trauma
- Allergies
- Infection
- Tumour
- Tongue

Box 4.3 Causes of external obstruction (upper airway)

- Soft tissue swelling in the neck due to haematoma, oedema, surgical emphysema (air in the tissues)
- Tumours in the neck
- Thyroid gland enlargement
- Cervical lymphadenopathy (swollen glands in the neck)

Reflection Points

1. *If the onset of airway obstruction is sudden and the patient has been well until then, what are the most likely causes?*
   Is it likely that the patient has either inhaled a foreign body such as a coin, peanut or has choked on food? There is also the possibility of an acute anaphylactic reaction causing severe upper airway oedema.
2. *If the patient has been feverish, and complains of a sore throat or hoarseness prior to the onset of airway obstruction what are the most likely causes?*
   Acute epiglottitis, tonsillitis or diphtheria may have caused this.

---

back slaps and abdominal thrusts (the Heimlich manoeuvre). This is an emergency situation and you should call for help using the emergency buzzer or calling out. Management should follow UK Resuscitation Council guidelines (2006).

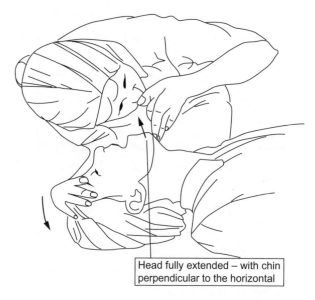

Head fully extended – with chin perpendicular to the horizontal

Fig. 4.2 Head tilt/chin lift

Manually opening the airway

1. If the patient is on their back, use either the head tilt/chin lift technique or the jaw thrust if there is any suspicion of neck trauma.
2. Inspect the mouth and pharynx for visible obstructions (mucus, food, foreign bodies).
3. If there is a visible obstruction that can be removed without forcing it further down the airway, then use suction or McGill's forceps to extract it. Only use suction on what you can see.
4. If the patient is unable to maintain their own airway due to reduced consciousness, consider placing an airway adjunct. The type of airway used will depend on how deeply uncon- scious the patient is. If there is any likelihood that they may gag and/or vomit then an oropharyngeal airway should not be used and a nasopharyngeal airway placed instead. If the patient is deeply unconscious (Glasgow Coma Scale score less

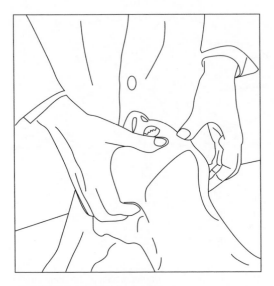

Fig. 4.3 Jaw thrust manoeuvre used where there is suspicion of neck trauma

than 9 or only responding to pain on the AVPU scale), then a definitive airway such as a laryngeal mask airway or an endotracheal tube will be needed. The patient will require oxygen via a mask with reservoir bag to ensure high levels of oxygen are delivered.

Oropharyngeal (Guedel) airway

Oropharyngeal (Guedel) airways are curved rigid plastic tubes with a flange, reinforced bite block and a curved flattened oval length of hollow plastic (Figure 4.4). They come in a range of sizes varying in length from 5 to 10 cm. The most common sizes used for adults are size 3 and 4, although large adults may require a 5. The correct size is determined by measuring the airway against the patient's face (Roberts and Porter 2003). The flange is placed at the patient's incisors and the correct size airway will the end at the angle of the jaw.

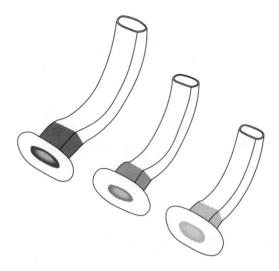

Fig. 4.4 Oropharyngeal (Guedel) airway

The airway is initially placed in the mouth with the curve facing upwards, but as soon as the end is past the hard palate the airway is rotated 180° allowing it to fit over the base of the tongue, thus bringing the tongue forward off the back of the pharynx. If the patient shows any sign of gagging or resisting the airway, remove it at once.

The lumen of the airway allows access to suction the upper airway, although the size of the suction catheter that can be used is limited.

Nasopharyngeal airway (NPA)

These are round curved plastic tubes bevelled at one end and with a flange at the other (Figure 4.5). They are usually made from latex, PVC or silicone and are softer than oropharyngeal airways. Size varies from a 6.0 mm to 9.0 mm internal diameter. When placed through the nostril, the NPA should sit approximately 10 mm above the epiglottis. Recommendations based on studies

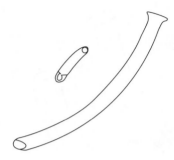

Fig. 4.5 Nasopharyngeal airway

of average nasopharyngeal airway length suggest that the size used should be related to height (Roberts et al, 2005). Therefore a woman of average height (around 5 ft 4 in, 1.62 m) should have a size 6.0 mm (length 130 mm) NPA and an average height man (around 5 ft 10 ins, 1.77 m) should have a size 7.0 mm (length 150 mm) NPA. Taller than average men will require a size 8 NPA.

Placing a nasopharyngeal airway

The nostrils should be visualised to identify any blockage and the right nostril should be tried first; however, if any blockage is seen or any resistance is encountered then the left nostril should be used. The airway is lubricated with water-soluble lubricant and placed bevel end down into the nostril. It is manoeuvred in along the floor of the nostril by keeping the bevel in the horizontal plane as it encounters the back of the pharynx. Gentle twisting may help to manoeuvre the NPA round the curve into the nasopharynx.

Some NPAs have safety pins to ensure that they do not slip down the nose and this should be applied before inserting the NPA into the nostril. Other types of NPA have an incorporated swivel safety grip which prevents slippage.

The nasopharyngeal airway is a useful adjunct which should always be considered when there is doubt about the ability of the patient to maintain their own airway but there is still evidence of gag reflex and resistance.

Key Point

Caution with NPAs

1. Suspicion of a basal skull fracture – the NPA may be misplaced into the brain via the skull fracture.
2. Coagulopathy – the lining of the nasal passages is very vascular, bleeding easily and copiously in a patient with poor clotting function. This will add to the problems of maintaining an airway in a semi-conscious patient.

Suction to clear the airway

When patients are unable to cough or to swallow secretions, saliva and sputum, then suction will be needed to assist clearance of the airway. Suction techniques are an essential skill and all nurses should be capable of oral suction and preferably tracheal suction too.

Safety principles for suctioning

Suction pressure should not be set above 26 kPa (200 mmHg) for oral suction and should be set between 13 and 16 kPa (100–170 mmHg) for tracheal suction.

If the patient has borderline hypoxaemia (oxygen saturations are <90%), then additional oxygen should be given prior to commencing suction. The amount of extra oxygen given will depend on how much the patient is already receiving.

No more than four suction catheters should be passed without allowing the patient time to recover. Pulse oximetry should continue during suction. Oral suction will require a Yankauer sucker, which is a wide bore rigid plastic sucker with multiple holes at the rounded end. This can only be used in the oropharyngeal cavity and should be inserted with care and moved from one side to the other in order to clear any secretions. Gloves and eye/face protection are worn to protect the user.

Nasopharyngeal and tracheal suction will require the use of sterile multi-eyed suction catheters with inbuilt suction control.

Suction technique

1. Prior to commencing suction, the patient should be told what will happen.
2. All necessary equipment (Box 4.4) should be checked, hands washed and protective equipment or clothing put on.

Box 4.4 Equipment list for suction

- Vacuum source (usually wall-mounted in hospital but may also be portable). Should have adjustable pressure regulator and filter.
- Collection reservoir and disposable tubing.
- Yankauer sucker or sterile multiple-eye suction catheters sized appropriately (i.e. size 8 to 10 for NPA and size 12 to 14 for oropharyngeal airway).
- Sterile disposable gloves.
- Sterile water for clearing tubing (when opened, it must be dated and timed).
- Clean disposable gloves.
- Apron.
- Goggles or visor for eye/face protection
- Water-soluble lubricant (sterile) for NPA suction.
- Oxygen delivery system and pulse oximeter. (Adam and Osborne 2005).

---

3. The number of sterile suction catheters thought to be needed (not usually more than four) are opened at one end onto the trolley and also the same number of single sterile or clean gloves. Soluble lubricant is also opened.
4. Suction is set to the correct level and the tubing is tucked under one arm with the connector readily available.
5. Alcohol hand gel is applied and a pair of clean gloves put on. (This is to protect the user.)
6. The sterile/clean glove is applied to the right hand (if right handed) and the suction catheter connecting end is picked up with the sterile/clean gloved hand and pushed into the tubing connector.

7. The rest of the packaging is slid off the suction catheter with the sterile/clean gloved hand controlling the process so that the end of the catheter does not flick into an unsterile area.
8. If using lubricant, the end of the catheter is smeared with the lubricant.
9. The patient is alerted that the suction catheter is about to enter the nasopharyngeal or tracheal airway and the suction catheter is guided into the airway.
10. The suction catheter is advanced until resistance is met or until the patient starts to cough. (If the suction catheter meets resistance but is not in far enough, then attempt to rotate slightly in order to continue advancing.)
11. Once in the right place, the left thumb is placed over the suction control and the catheter is withdrawn smoothly (no rotation) with suction maintained throughout.
12. The whole process should not take more than around 30 seconds, with suction itself lasting between 10 and 15 seconds.
13. The suction catheter is removed and rolled round the sterile/ clean glove on the right hand. This is then slid off over the top of the catheter so that the catheter is contained within the glove. These items can then be disposed of in clinical waste.
14. Once suctioning is complete, the tubing should be rinsed through with sterile water.

Remember: some patients may have a permanent tracheostomy – this is the patient's airway. Clear the stoma using suction and ensure that any method of oxygen delivery is placed over the stoma rather than over the mouth and nose.

SUMMARY

Airway assessment is the most vital part of any assessment. All nurses should be capable of identifying when a patient's airway is compromised (i.e. it is either partially or completely obstructed). Partial obstruction is characterised by increased sounds associated with the movement of air through narrowed airways but complete obstruction will have little or no increased sounds as there is no air movement. The patient will be extremely agitated and will rapidly become grey/blue in colour. Partial obstruction can be caused by a number of factors both inside and outside the airway itself. Maintaining the patency of the patient's airway requires a range of techniques from back-slapping and the Heimlich manoeuvre to suction. Any form of airway obstruction should be regarded as an emergency and if interventions such as suction cannot immediately clear the problem, then expert help should be called immediately.

CLINICAL SCENARIOS

Scenario 4.1

You are caring for a patient who has recently been admitted with non-Hodgkin's Lymphoma (malignant lymphocytic disease). He has gross cervical lymphadenopathy (swelling of the lymph glands in the neck) and complains that he has been unable to eat food or sleep properly recently.

Q1 What would you assess?

The patient's respiratory rate is 25 breaths/minute and his SpO_2 is 93%. His temperature is 36.5°C and his pulse is 110bpm. His blood pressure is 135/90mmHg. He has a whispery voice and he is unable to cough properly. His air entry is reduced throughout the chest and there are coarse crackles at the bases. When you attempt to lay him flat, he becomes very distressed and requests to be sat upright.

Q2 What would you do?

After the doctor has seen him and prescribed 40% humidified oxygen and intravenous hydrocortisone, the patient complains of difficulty swallowing his saliva and can hardly get his words out. His respiratory rate is now 30 breaths/minute and SpO_2 is 92% on 40% humidified oxygen.

Q3 What should you do now?

Answers to scenario 4.1

1. A – The patient is unable to speak at normal volume or cough and he hasn't been able to swallow food. These are all features of a threatened or partially obstructed airway from his neck swelling.

   B – Respiratory rate – and oxygen saturations – should be measured and air entry auscultated. It is likely that the patient has been unable to clear his chest secretions as he cannot cough properly and these will collect causing further respiratory compromise and potential infection.

   C – Pulse rate, blood pressure, temperature and capillary refill time should be monitored.

   D – The patient is talking and is orientated.

   E – Neck swelling is bilateral and the patient's mouth is very dry.

2. The patient should have warmed/humidified oxygen (humidified to reduce further trauma to the mucosa from dry gas which would increase swelling). The patient should be sat upright. The doctor should be informed at once. Critical care outreach and the anaesthetist should be called to advise on the need for a pre-emptive tracheostomy to ensure the airway is protected (it would be very difficult to perform an emergency intubatation in a patient with this degree of neck swelling).

3. An anaesthetist should be called urgently to support the patient's airway and an ENT surgeon or intensive care consultant (because they are able to perform a tracheostomy) should also be called urgently. A tracheostomy should be urgently considered. The patient should be moved to a high dependency area where his airway can be closely monitored. Steroids should be given to reduce the level of swelling in the neck. Intravenous fluids should be commenced as the patient is likely to be dehydrated.

Scenario 4.2

You are taking over on the night shift and as you approach one of the recent post-operative patients on your ward to check the patient-controlled analgesia you hear slow, gurgling snoring from the patient, who is lying on his back. The last time the observations were done on this patient was over 2 hours ago. The patient has an intravenous infusion of 0.9% saline running.

Q1 What would you assess?

The patient's snoring improves with a head tilt/chin lift manoeuvre and you place them in the recovery position. The patient is unresponsive and the respiratory rate is only 6 breaths/minute. The SpO_2 is 92% on 2 l/min oxygen via nasal cannulae. The PCA analgesia is fentanyl, which is a synthetic opiate. Pulse rate is 90 bpm with a moderate pulse volume and blood pressure is 94/60 mmHg (previously 128/80 mmHg). Temperature is 37°C. CRT is 2 seconds. Pupils are pinpoint (size 2 mm) and reactions to light are difficult to assess.

Q2 What would you do now?

The doctor arrives and prescribes 0.8 mg of naloxone intravenously. Following administration of the naloxone the patient begins to respond and respiratory rate increases to 12 breaths/minute. Arterial blood gas shows a pCO_2 of 6.8 kPa and pO_2 of 9.7 kPa.

Q3 What is the ongoing care needed for this patient?

Answers to scenario 4.2

1. A – The patient's airway is compromised. Check the tongue is not obstructing the airway by either waking the patient (if this is possible) and getting them to move on to their side or by applying head tilt/chin lift manoeuvre to see if this opens the airway.

   B – Respiratory rate and saturations.

C – Pulse, blood pressure, temperature, capillary refill time.
D – Responsiveness, pupil size and reaction to light.

2. Place a facemask delivering oxygen at 35% on the patient and call for help. Stop the analgesia. Call the doctor and critical care outreach if available. Check suction is available. Ensure the patient remains in the recovery position and remain with them.

   It is likely that naloxone will be needed to reverse the opiate. Ask one of the staff to ensure it is available.

3. Naloxone has a fairly short period of effectiveness and the patient may become drowsy once more. Frequent (15 minute) observations are required of conscious level, respiratory rate and SpO_2 until the effects of the opiate have worn off and the patient is stable.

   Pain levels should also be assessed frequently as the naloxone will counteract the analgesic effect of the opiate.

Scenario 4.3

You are looking after the ward during the evening meal and you see that an elderly lady has gone very red in the face and is gesticulating at you and holding her neck. As you approach she becomes more agitated and you see that she is making enormous effort to breathe.

Q1 What do you think has happened?

Q2 What would you do?

After you have attempted to clear the obstruction using the Heimlich manoeuvre, her eyes roll up and she slumps back in the bed.

The staff nurse brings the ward emergency trolley, and you are able clear the patient's mouth with suction. You should not suction further than you can see, as it is possible to push any foreign body further into the airway. The cardiac arrest team arrive and the anaesthetist attempts to view the vocal cords with the laryngoscope.

Answers to scenario 4.3

1. The patient has inhaled some of her supper and is choking on it.
2. Pull the arrest buzzer and call for help. If the patient is still conscious, lean her forward and apply five sharp blows to the back, checking whether this has worked between each blow. If the patient loses consciousness, start basic life support with a bag valve mask and 100% oxygen.

REFERENCES AND FURTHER READING

Adam SK, Osborne S (2005) Critical Care Nursing: Science and practice. Oxford University Press, Oxford

Resuscitation Council UK (2006) Advanced Life Support (5th edn). UK Resuscitation Council, London

Roberts K, Porter K (2003) How do you size a nasopharyngeal airway? Resuscitation 56:19–23

Roberts K, Whalley H, Bleetman A (2005) The nasopharyngeal airway: dispelling myths and establishing the facts. Emergency Medical Journal 22:394–396

Smith G (2000) ALERT™ A multiprofessional course in care of the acutely ill patient. The Open Learning Centre, University of Portsmouth

---

Answers to Learning Points

1. Is it likely that the patient has either inhaled a foreign body such as a coin, peanut or has choked on food? There is also the possibility of an acute anaphylactic reaction causing severe upper airway oedema.
2. Acute epiglottitis, tonsillitis or diphtheria may have caused this.

A-**B**-C-D-E: Breathing (and Failure to Breathe)

5

INTRODUCTION

The most important issues to consider during patient assessment are whether or not there is enough oxygen being taken into the lungs and then whether or not that oxygen is being delivered to the tissues in sufficient quantities; i.e., breathing and circulation are very much interlinked.

Breathing involves the taking in of oxygen to the lungs where it diffuses into the circulatory system for transport throughout the body, and also the removal of waste carbon dioxide generated by cellular metabolism. Without sufficient oxygen, body organs cannot function properly and may be irreversibly damaged within a few minutes, while insufficient elimination of carbon dioxide allows toxic levels to accumulate.

The recent *Burden of Lung Disease* report details the scale of acute and chronic respiratory disease in the UK (British Thoracic Society, 2006). For example:

- There were 554,921 emergency admissions to English hospitals in 2004–2005 due to respiratory disease, making it the second most common cause of emergency admission (after injury and poisoning).
- Patients with respiratory disease used over 5.2 million hospital bed days in 2004–2005; mostly for treatment of acute lower respiratory tract infections (pneumonia, influenza etc.) and chronic obstructive lung disease.
- Respiratory disease kills one in five people in the UK (117,456 deaths in 2004).

Issues around the assessment of upper airway patency and the first-line management of an obstructed airway have been discussed in the previous chapter. This chapter provides an overview of the important physiological processes in respiration, outlines a systematic approach to the assessment of breathing and how common problems can be recognised, and how key treatments may be used – in particular, the giving of oxygen. The analysis of arterial blood gases is discussed in Appendix 1: Acid–base balance and arterial blood gases.

LEARNING OBJECTIVES
By the end of this chapter you should be able to:

❏ Understand the physiological processes involved in getting oxygen into the circulation, and in expelling carbon dioxide
❏ Describe signs, symptoms and common causes of acute respiratory failure
❏ Detail a systematic approach to rapid assessment of breathing
❏ Outline how oxygenation can be effectively monitored in a ward area
❏ Discuss the indications for oxygen therapy – and the appropriate oxygen delivery system for different situations
❏ Understand when expert help may be needed.

ANATOMY AND PHYSIOLOGY REFRESHER
The respiratory tract consists of the upper airways, trachea, bronchi, and lungs (see Figure 5.1). An understanding of the route by which air enters and moves through the body is essential, and can also help the practitioner work out the nature of any breathing problems. That is, for example, there may be a blockage of some kind in the upper airways (e.g. due to the tongue falling back in the pharynx or inhalation of a foreign object) or constriction of the bronchi (e.g. in asthma or chronic obstructive pulmonary disease) or infection or fluid in the alveoli of the lungs. Thinking in turn about each of these components of the respiratory tract can guide a systematic assessment.

Trachea and bronchi
The trachea connects to the larynx at its upper end and at its lower end divides into the right and left main bronchi, which enter the right and left lung respectively. The bronchi branch from the trachea and then repeatedly subdivide throughout the lungs.

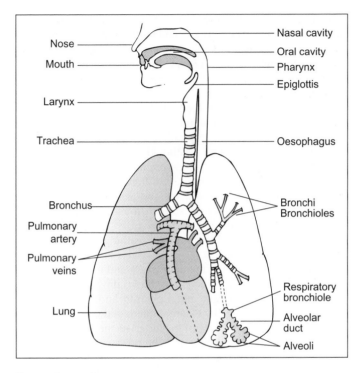

Fig. 5.1 The respiratory system
From Petersen O, Lecture Notes: Human Physiology (5th edn), copyright 2006 with permission of Blackwell Publishing Ltd

The lungs

The lungs are two large cone shaped organs situated either side of the heart and occupying most of the chest. Each lung is surrounded by a double-layered pleural membrane, which is attached to the internal surfaces of the chest wall, the diaphragm and structures in the mediastinum. The lungs enclose the bronchi and their many divisions, the smallest of which are termed bronchioles. The bronchioles lead to alveoli (air sacs) where oxygen diffuses across the alveolar wall into a fine network of pulmonary capillaries and carbon dioxide diffuses from capillaries into the alveoli for exhalation. There are approximately 300 million alveoli in the lung, in a respiratory membrane (or pulmonary membrane) up to $100\,m^2$ in area through which oxygen and carbon dioxide can be exchanged (West, 2004).

Breathing

Normally, the rate and depth of breathing are regulated without conscious effort by the autonomic nervous system. Nervous stimulation of the muscles of respiration is primarily controlled by structures in the brainstem – although other parts of the brain can also have an influence. These brainstem structures work in response to input from a system of different sensors that detect changes in oxygen, carbon dioxide and acid levels in the body, and also sense the tension in smooth muscles in the airways. Elevated carbon dioxide and acid or reduced oxygen in cerebral spinal fluid or blood tend to stimulate breathing, while distension of the lungs slows it down.

Inspiration occurs when the diaphragm and external intercostal muscles contract. The lungs are drawn downwards by contraction of the diaphragm and upwards and forwards with expansion of the ribcage by external intercostal contraction. This process increases the volume of the lungs, so that the residual air inside occupies a larger space and the pressure exerted by that air is reduced. Air in the atmosphere is at a similar pressure to air in the lungs before inspiration occurs, but when the pressure in the lungs decreases, atmospheric air moves into the lungs (i.e. from an area of relatively higher pressure to one of lower pressure) until the pressures in the lungs equilibrate with atmospheric pressure. In expiration, the respiratory muscles relax and the elastic quality of the lungs brings them back to their resting position. This raises the pressure in the lungs relative to the atmosphere, and forces air out until pressures in the lungs equilibrate with atmospheric pressure once more (Box 5.1).

Box 5.1 How oxygen gets into the circulation

Getting oxygen into the circulation depends on three main factors (created from West 2004):

1. Firstly, the lung volume, which correlates with the area of respiratory membrane available for gaseous exchange:
   - Simply changing position from a flat-lying to a sitting position can increase lung volume by about 40%, enabling significantly more gaseous exchange to occur. Note also that a large or distended abdomen may compress the chest cavity, particularly if the patient is lying flat. If abdominal distension is caused by excessive air or fluid in the stomach, a nasogastric tube can be used to decompress the stomach and enable easier respiration.
   - Excessive fluid or mucus in the lungs, or collapse of areas of lung tissue (e.g. due to blockage of bronchi and bronchioles, or air, fluid, blood or pus within the pleural membranes) may all reduce the lung volume available for gaseous exchange.
2. Secondly, the amount of oxygen in the air in the alveoli relative to amounts in the pulmonary capillaries.
   - In a healthy young adult breathing air, there is typically about 14 kPa of oxygen in the alveolus, and 5–6 kPa of oxygen dissolved in the venous blood within the pulmonary capillary approaching the alveolus (Oh, 2003). Oxygen in the alveolus will move from an area of relatively higher concentration to one of lower concentration in the capillary until the levels are more or less the same (capillary oxygen rising to, say, 13 kPa) – within a fraction of a second.
   - With oxygen therapy, the amount of oxygen in the alveoli can be increased and therefore so can the size of the concentration gradient and the amount that diffuses into the circulation.
   - Note that hypoventilation (reduced rate or depth of breathing) allows carbon dioxide to accumulate in the alveoli (rather than being exhaled), which leaves less room for oxygen. This will tend to reduce the amount of oxygen available for movement into the circulation.
3. Thirdly, the thickness of the tissue between the alveoli and capillaries. This is normally less than one-thousandth of a millimetre, but it increases with age and in acute and chronic respiratory diseases so that gaseous exchange is hindered (e.g., with infection or inflammation, or fibrosis of the alveoli and interstitial tissues of the lungs).

It is useful to consider two other issues – if possible. (These may be assessed more thoroughly during examination of the circulatory system.)

- The blood can only be oxygenated when there is an adequate flow of blood through the pulmonary circulation. However, if the flow is reduced (e.g. because blood volume is low, or there is obstruction by pulmonary emboli), it is less likely that sufficient oxygen can be transported to the tissues. Oxygen in alveoli adjacent to capillaries with low blood flows is essentially wasted oxygen. Similarly, blood in capillaries adjacent to alveoli that do not contain oxygen (because they are blocked or collapsed) is wasted blood. These situations are instances of ventilation/perfusion mismatch.

- Once oxygen enters the blood stream, it usually rapidly attaches to whatever haemoglobin is present; indeed, oxygen is largely transported in the circulation bound to haemoglobin (1 g of haemoglobin carries about 1.36 ml of oxygen when it is 100% saturated). This means that the quantity of oxygen delivered to the tissues is a function of Hb levels in the circulation, how saturated that Hb is with oxygen and the amount of blood flow. (The theory and practice of assessing blood flow are discussed in the next chapter.)

Consider two patients, both of a similar size, with similar cardiovascular function (e.g., each pumping about 5 litres of blood per minute) and both with Hb in the normal range (13.5–17.5 g/dl). Think about which of these patients is likely to have more oxygen circulating through the body.

Mr Smith has an Hb of 14, and oxygen saturation 99%, while Mr Jones has an Hb of 17, and an oxygen saturation of only 85%. Which is better?

$$\text{Oxygen delivery} = \text{cardiac output in l/min}$$
$$[5 \text{ l/min for both patients in this example}]$$
$$\times \text{Hb concentration (g/dl)} \times 1.36 \text{ (ml } O_2/\text{g Hb)}$$
$$\times \% \text{ oxygen saturation}$$

- Smith has an oxygen delivery of $5 \times 14 \times 1.36 \times 99 = 9425$ ml of oxygen delivered per minute;
- Jones' oxygen delivery is $5 \times 17 \times 1.36 \times 85 = 9826$ ml of oxygen delivered per minute – *more than Smith.*

These sorts of calculations are not often performed in ward settings, but the principles are useful. For example, patients with chronic obstructive lung diseases often have a compensatory polycythaemia (raised red blood cell and haemoglobin levels); if this is the case, it may be that they can be managed with relatively lower oxygen saturations – as long as they carefully monitored. In contrast, anaemic patients are not easily able to transport sufficient oxygen to the tissues, so oxygen saturations will probably need to be maximised – and the adequacy of blood flow assessed – to ensure that there is enough oxygen in the system.

Note: Even if a patient with low oxygen saturation has high haemoglobin, it does not mean that they are stable. 85% oxygen saturation for any significant length of time *is* very low: the patient either has a severe acute illness or a serious – perhaps end-stage – chronic disease. A further reduction in oxygen saturation could well be life-threatening: a decrease from 100% to 95% may indicate a new problem but is not in itself dangerous, but a drop from 85% to 80% is a high-risk event.

OXYGENATION OF THE BLOOD

Oxygen in the blood is found in two forms.

1. When oxygen diffuses into the capillary from the alveolus it may immediately encounter a red blood cell and attach to the cell's haemoglobin. Each molecule of haemoglobin can hold up to four oxygen molecules. If three oxygen molecules are attached to one molecule of haemoglobin molecule it is three-quarters or 75% saturated. If there are four oxygen molecules, the haemoglobin is 100% saturated. Oxygen saturation measured by a pulse oximeter averages the saturation of the large number of haemoglobin molecules in the circulation (see Box 5.2).

2. Usually, at least 98% of the oxygen in the blood is attached to haemoglobin (which is why haemoglobin is so important), leaving a small amount dissolved in plasma. This dissolved oxygen is still significant because the more oxygen there is in solution, the more likely it is that every haemoglobin molecule can become saturated. The molecules of a dissolved gas create what is called tension – or pressure – in the solution: the more that is dissolved, the higher the pressure. The pressure created by oxygen

(and carbon dioxide) dissolved in the plasma can be measured by analysis of a sample of arterial blood (arterial blood gas).

The relationship between the pressure of oxygen dissolved in the plasma (pO_2) and the saturation of haemoglobin (SaO_2) is shown in Figures 5.2 and 5.3. The more or less s-shaped curve in Figure 5.3 is known as the oxygen dissociation curve or the oxyhaemoglobin dissociation curve (oxyhaemoglobin is haemoglobin with oxygen attached). It can be seen that in the upper, flatter part of the curve, increases in pO_2 only produce a marginal increase in saturation; but lower down on the steeper section of the curve, a relatively small reduction in pO_2 results in a significant fall in saturation. For example, adding another 2.6 kPa of dissolved oxygen to a pO_2 of 8.0 kPa increases the SaO_2 from 90 to 95%, but taking 2.6 kPa of oxygen from a level of 8.0 kPa leads to a life-threatening drop in SaO_2 to about 75%.

It should be noted that particular pO_2 values do not correspond exactly with specific saturations all the time: the relationship is affected by several factors including changes in temperature and acid levels in the body. However, as a rule, the higher the pressure of oxygen dissolved in the blood, the higher the oxygen saturation of haemoglobin.

Measuring oxygenation

The oxygen content of the blood can be assessed in two ways. The first is by using a pulse oximeter to measure arterial oxygen saturation (SaO_2), i.e. the percentage of circulating haemoglobin that is saturated with oxygen.

Pressure of O_2 in plasma (pO_2) (in kPa)	13.3	12.9	10.6	9.3	8.0	6.7	5.3	4.0
						hypoxia		
Percentage Hb saturated with O_2 (SaO_2)	99	97	95	93	90	85	75	60

Fig. 5.2 Relationship between oxygen tension and percentage of haemoglobin saturated with oxygen in arterial blood
Adapted from Oh (2003)

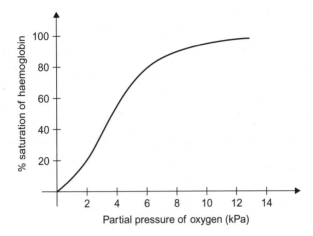

Fig. 5.3 Oxygen dissociation curve: the higher the pressure of oxygen dissolved in plasma (pO_2), measured in kPa, the higher the % saturation of haemoglobin
From Esmond G, Mikelsons C, Non-Invasive Respiratory Support Techniques, copyright 2008 with permission of Wiley-Blackwell

---

Box 5.2 The Pulse Oximeter

The pulse oximeter probe is usually placed on a finger, toe or earlobe. The device emits red and infrared light, some of which is absorbed by haemoglobin in the tissue beneath. It can also put pressure on the tissue and generate some heat, which has occasionally been reported to cause tissue damage. Therefore the probe should be moved to a new site every 2 hours or so. The pattern of light absorption varies depending on whether or not the haemoglobin has oxygen attached to it, and a sensor in the probe can detect these different patterns. The device is also able to differentiate between arterial and venous blood, and then calculate how much of the haemoglobin in arterial blood has oxygen attached to it, which it displays as a percentage value (SpO_2).

The key points in oximetry are (McMorrow and Mythen, 2006):

- The pulse oximeter will only function if there is an adequate flow of blood through the site being employed, and if the site is reasonably still (which means it can be difficult to use on a restless

Box 5.2 (cont'd)

patient). Some machines display the signal strength which helps show whether or not sufficient blood flow is present. If the oximeter does not seem to be working properly, it is worth trying different sites for the probe, such as the earlobe. The practitioner can also test it on his or her own finger. If it works on you but is not working on the patient, it may be that the patient is in circulatory failure. Never assume that it is the machine that is faulty – it may be the patient that has the problem.

- Dark coloured nail varnish interferes with the light signal and should be removed from any digits used.
- The oximeter is designed to work with normal haemogloblin. Abnormal forms such as methaemoglobin (which cannot bind with oxygen) or haemoglobin in sickle cell disease give false readings. Carboxyhaemoglobin – found in cases of carbon monoxide poisoning – causes inaccuracies too.
- Some substances used as intravenous dyes and for other purposes (e.g. methylene blue, indocyanine green) can cause a false SpO_2.
- Bright daylight or fluorescent lighting may also cause inaccuracies.

Note: Strictly speaking, oxygen saturation measured from a sample of arterial blood is labelled as SaO_2 (the 'a' indicates the arterial component), while oxygen saturation measured with a pulse oximeter is SpO_2, the 'p' denoting pulse oximetry.

Key Point

The British Thoracic Society suggest the following target oxygen saturations in acute illness (O'Driscoll et al, 2008):

- 94–98% for most patients
- 88–92% for patients at risk of hypercapnic respiratory failure – that is, those with chronically raised carbon dioxide levels (e.g. with chronic obstructive pulmonary disease, morbid obesity, chest wall deformities or neuromuscular disorders).

Supplementary oxygen should be given to the acutely ill hypoxaemic patient to achieve the appropriate target saturation for that individual, generally by using a high concentration mask with non-rebreathe reservoir bag and oxygen flow ≥10 l/min. (O'Driscoll et al, 2008).

The second way oxygen content of the blood can be appraised is by sampling arterial blood – usually termed arterial blood gas analysis – to measure the pO_2. The pO_2 of inspired air (containing 21% oxygen) is approximately 20.0 kPa, but this falls by about a third to around 14 kPa by the time it reaches the alveolus (of a healthy young adult), and by a little more once diffused into the circulation – giving, say, an arterial pO_2 of 13 kPa (and perhaps a SaO_2 of 99%). The pO_2 value tends to reduce with age – even in healthy individuals – so it may be 12.0 kPa in those aged 60 years, and 11.0 kPa in 80 year olds.

Key Question 1

Is there enough oxygen in the blood?

(remembering that there also needs to be enough Hb in the blood)
Hypoxaemia can be defined as pO_2 <8 kPa or SaO_2 <90% (O'Driscoll et al, 2008).

The effects of oxygen therapy and the alveolar–arterial oxygen gradient

It was shown above that when breathing room air – which has a 21% oxygen content (approximately equal to 20.0 kPa), a healthy adult will end up with 11.0–13.3 kPa in his or her blood. In other words, there is normally a gradient or gap of roughly 10.0 kPa between the amount of oxygen inspired and the arterial pO_2 (in kPa). Because the percentage of oxygen in air is not much different to the pressure in kPa, the simplest way of thinking about this gap is just to subtract the pO_2 obtained from an arterial blood sample from the percentage of inspired oxygen (whatever that might be: e.g., 21%, 50%, or 100% oxygen). This means that if 100% oxygen is inspired, it may be expected that there will be <90 kPa in the blood of a healthy young adult; breathing 50% oxygen will give about 40 kPa in the blood; and so on.

However, if the gap between the amount of oxygen inspired (as a percentage) and the oxygen in the blood (in kPa) is much more than 10, it suggests that there is either a problem with oxygen getting into the alveoli in the first place or that the oxygen cannot easily cross from the alveoli into the pulmonary circulation. That is, either the lung volume/area of respiratory membrane available for gaseous exchange is reduced (perhaps due to infection), or the tissue between alveoli and capillaries has thickened (perhaps due to oedema). A gap of more than 20 is indicative of a significant disease process. Of course, as long as the arterial pO_2 is >10–11 kPa, the oxygen saturation will probably still be in the normal range. But, if a normal pO_2 and SaO_2 can only be obtained by giving, say, more than 35% oxygen, it must be recognised that the patient is at risk or has an actual acute illness. If more than 50% oxygen is required, the patient is at high risk and/or has a serious illness. This means that it is essential that the percentage of inspired oxygen – or at least the oxygen flow in l/min – is recorded when pO_2 or oxygen saturation is measured. It is not always possible to determine the exact oxygen concentration delivered by a particular flow rate through nasal cannulae or most facemasks. The most commonly used oxygen administration devices, flow rates and approximate oxygen concentrations associated with those flow rates are given in Appendix 2, Oxygen delivery devices.

Key Point

Remember, as a general rule:

- If more than 35% oxygen is needed to achieve a normal pO_2 and SaO_2, the patient is *at risk* of deterioration.
- If more than 50% oxygen is needed to achieve a normal pO_2 and SaO_2, the patient is at *high risk* of deterioration.
- If the gap between the amount of inspired oxygen and the oxygen in the blood increases over time, *the patient is deteriorating*; or if an increasing amount of supplementary oxygen is needed to achieve a normal pO_2 and SaO_2, *the patient is deteriorating*.

CARBON DIOXIDE

The main functions of breathing are to supply the body with oxygen and to rid it of waste carbon dioxide (CO_2). Normal body metabolism continually produces CO_2 – typically, 15,000–

20,000 mmol/day. The hypermetabolism that often accompanies acute illness can significantly increase this amount. Consequently, there is always a baseline level of CO_2 in the blood – measured in terms of the tension or pressure it exerts – with a normal range of 4.6–6.1 kPa (O'Driscoll et al, 2008). CO_2 tends to combine with water in the body in a process that can generate excessive acid, which in turn has adverse effects on cellular metabolism throughout the body. Elevated CO_2 and acid levels will eventually depress consciousness and may even cause coma. Therefore it can be seen that there is a constant need for removal of carbon dioxide from the body. CO_2 levels in the blood correlate with the volumes of air exhaled. If the rate or depth of breathing is increased (hyperventilation), pCO_2 falls; but if individuals slow their breathing or hold their breath (hypoventilation) – even for a short time – pCO_2 (and acid) levels rise.

Key Question 2

Is breathing adequate to eliminate enough carbon dioxide?

The only way of being certain that the pCO_2 is in the normal range is to measure the level in an arterial blood sample. However, if the patient has a respiratory rate in the normal range (12–20) *and* there seems to be normal air entry to all areas of the lungs *and* there are no abnormal systemic signs – particularly reduced consciousness – it is likely (though not definite) that the pCO_2 is normal or near-normal. Even so, if the patient is presenting with a new acute respiratory illness or exacerbation of a chronic respiratory disorder, it is usually useful to analyse at least one set of arterial blood gases. A summary of arterial blood gas analysis and common acid, base, oxygen and carbon dioxide abnormalities can be found in Appendix 1.

SIGNS, SYMPTOMS AND CAUSES OF RESPIRATORY FAILURE

Failure to breathe adequately can conveniently be placed under two main headings, essentially defined by oxygen and carbon dioxide levels in the blood.

Type 1 respiratory failure

This occurs when the primary problem is hypoxaemia ($pO_2 < 8\,kPa$ or $SaO_2 < 90\%$) and the pCO_2 is not raised (the pCO_2 may even be low). Type 1 failure is most often due to an acute problem such as pneumonia or some other respiratory infection, acute asthma, excess fluid in the lung tissue (pulmonary oedema) and/or in the pleural membranes (pleural effusion), pulmonary embolism; or air, blood or pus within the pleural membranes (pneumothorax, haemothorax or empyema). Hypoxaemia can also occur even when the alveoli are well ventilated, if there is insufficient blood flow through the pulmonary circulation. This is one form of so-called ventilation/perfusion mismatch, the other form being when there is good blood flow through the lungs but the alveoli are not adequately ventilated.

Type 2 respiratory failure

This is characterised by hypoxaemia *and* hypercarbia (pCO_2 above $6.1\,kPa$). Patients with the sorts of acute problems listed as causes of Type 1 failure may develop Type 2 failure if they tire and their respiratory effort decreases (i.e. they hypoventilate). However, Type 2 failure is more often a consequence of the worsening of some long-term disease process, particularly chronic obstructive pulmonary disease (COPD). Neuromuscular or skeletal disorders that reduce the ability to expand the chest (e.g. motor neurone disease or kyphoscoliosis) and other problems such as morbid obesity where the enlarged abdomen reduces chest expansion may also cause Type 2 respiratory failure.

When a patient is identified with pCO_2 above $6.1\,kPa$, it is then essential to determine whether or not the raised CO_2 has led to a significant excess of acid in the blood. People with long-term hypercarbia (e.g. in COPD) have compensatory mechanisms that usually offset the hypercarbia and keep the body's acid–base balance more or less in the normal range. But, in acute exacerbations of such chronic diseases, pCO_2 can rise higher than is usual even for these individuals. The compensatory mechanisms generally take some days to adjust, so in the meantime the patient may have dangerous levels of acid in the blood – indicated by a relatively low pH value. The pH can be measured by analysis of the arterial blood sample used to calculate pO_2 and pCO_2. Hypercarbia causing the pH to fall below the normal 7.35–7.45 range (the lower the pH value, the more the blood is relatively acid, and a pH less than 7.35 indicates that there are abnormally high levels of acid in the blood) can be treated by non-invasive pressure supported ventilation (NIV) – used in some ward areas – when repositioning, controlled oxygen therapy, nebulised salbutamol and ipratroprium, physiotherapy, etc. prove unsuccessful. NIV is primarily used to treat acute Type 2 respiratory failure – particularly acute exacerbations of COPD – where increasing pCO_2 levels are causing the blood to become relatively acid, i.e. when the serum pH is <7.35 (British Thoracic Society, 2002; Royal College of Physicians et al, 2008). NIV may improve hypoxaemia, but most NIV systems are not designed to treat severe hypoxaemia. Importantly, this treatment is most likely to be effective if applied early.

Breathlessness

Breathlessness is a less objective sign, but is very significant. Breathlessness is usually associated with a tachypnoea (rapid breathing: that is, a respiratory rate >20 breaths/minute) but is also a subjective feeling of difficulty breathing, shortness of breath or effortful breathing. Some people breathe fast without seeming to be troubled by it. Nonetheless, tachypnoea and breathlessness are important early warning signs of a whole range of illnesses – very often the first signs.

The respiratory rate generally increases in respiratory disease, but also in cardiovascular disease (e.g. in heart failure), in systemic diseases such as sepsis (when both hypoxaemia and elevated levels of acid in the blood may trigger increased respirations), and in disorders of the central nervous system (particularly brain injuries – e.g. trauma, stroke, haemorrhage – that have an impact on the brainstem). The patient's affective state (mood or emotion) can also be a factor (e.g. hyperventilation may be related to anxiety).

More information can be gained from considering the context of the breathlessness (if the situation allows):

- *Is this a new problem?* For example, a sudden onset may be due to pulmonary embolism (check for deep vein thrombosis:

examine the calves for warm and swollen tender or painful areas), acute asthma, pneumothorax; acute exacerbation of heart failure, or acute coronary syndrome/myocardial infarction. Conditions such as pneumonia or pleural effusion more often develop over a number of hours or days.

- *Is the patient breathless at rest or just on exertion?*
- *Does the breathlessness get better or worse when lying down?* If it is worse when lying flat, it may indicate heart failure.
- *Is the breathlessness associated with recent exposure to an allergen?* For example, asthma or anaphylaxis – often also associated with bronchoconstriction, stridor, wheeze.
- *What other problems does the patient have?* For example, breathlessness associated with a feeling of tightness, heaviness or pain in the chest may have a cardiac cause.

Systemic signs

The respiratory system does not exist in isolation from other body systems, and is especially interconnected with the cardiovascular system. This is illustrated by the 'CURB-65' assessment tool, which gives a score to patients presenting with community acquired pneumonia that helps show whether or not they need to be admitted to hospital, and, if so, whether admission to a ward or a critical care bed is needed.

Note that only one of these factors is obviously linked to respiratory function. Each factor identified scores 1, with a score of 3 or more indicating patients at high risk of death (British Thoracic Society, 2004).

- **C**onfusion
- **U**rea >7 mmol/l
- **R**espiratory rate ≥30/min
- Low systolic (<90 mmHg) or diastolic (≤60 mmHg) **B**lood pressure
- age ≥**65** years.

The CURB-65 system illustrates that a chest infection can have complications in terms of cardiovascular function (blood pressure), as well as brain function (new confusion), and renal function (serum urea). The more complications there are, the worse the patient outcome is likely to be.

Knowing the patient

A knowledge of the patient's medical history and hospital admission helps put any signs and symptoms of illness in context. New breathlessness and tachypnoea may have a number of causes, but review of the individual's background can help define the diagnosis. For example, there are known risk factors for pulmonary embolism – not least hospitalisation and immobility (e.g. recent abdominal or pelvic surgery, lower limb or joint fractures or surgery, pregnancy, malignant disease, etc.).

ASSESSMENT OF BREATHING

The *minimum* requirement is to:

- **Look** at – and talk to – the patient. **Look** for chest movement (rate, pattern, depth, symmetry, and effort).
- **Listen** to the patient response. **Listen** to breath sounds.
- **Measure** respiratory rate and oxygen saturation; and to consider whether or not it may be necessary to measure carbon dioxide levels.

Key Point

If at any stage it is obvious that the patient is showing signs of critical illness, administer high concentration oxygen via a face mask without delay (oxygen flow ≥10 l/min, using a mask with non-rebreathe reservoir bag if possible), and consider the need for urgent expert help.

On first approach

Introduce yourself and say what you plan to do (i.e. perform an assessment). Ask 'how are you?'

 **Look at the patient**

- What is his general appearance? Does he seem unwell, e.g. restless, agitated – or difficult to rouse? Does he seem to be in pain – and if so, is it directly associated to breathing?

- Are there any immediately obvious abnormalities?

It is usually worth helping the patient into a reasonably upright position if it appears that there is any difficulty breathing. This also makes it easier to properly assess the patient.

- Is the patient pale or flushed; or dusky, grey or blue (possible indicators of inadequate oxygenation or insufficient elimination of carbon dioxide); or sweaty?

  Hypoxaemia can cause vasoconstriction, and pallor. However, severe hypoxaemia can cause cyanosis. Make a point of looking at the lips (and tongue if possible). Blue lips and tongue (central cyanosis) indicate a serious and very possibly life-threatening respiratory or cardiovascular problem. Central cyanosis occurs when >5 g/dl of haemaglobin does not have oxygen attached: this would represent more than one-third of haemaglobin not saturated in someone with a normal Hb of 15 g/dl and is therefore a sign of a serious deficiency. High concentration supplemental oxygen should be started if not already in place. Alternatively, hypercarbia can cause vasodilation and flushing.

- Now look at the chest and chest movement (rate, pattern, depth, symmetry – and effort).
  - It is sometimes quite difficult to see chest movement in normal quiet breathing; but fortunately (!) patients in respiratory distress usually have quite obvious movement. If breathing is difficult to discern – and particularly if the patient is unresponsive – it may be that you are in a peri-respiratory arrest situation and need to call the resuscitation team (although such a state should have already been identified in the initial assessment/assessment of airway patency stage).
  - Even without exact counting, it is usually easy to gauge whether the respiratory rate is fast, slow or normal (12–20 breaths/minute). Slow breathing has a potential to cause hypercarbia – the pCO_2 in an arterial blood sample may need to be checked in due course, particularly if the patient is drowsy. Fast breathing may be a sign of an acute respiratory problem, but also of cardiovascular or systemic disease, and is usually tiring for the patient. A prolonged respiratory rate

of ≥25 breaths/minute is indicative of a patient at significant risk of deterioration.

– Check the pattern or rhythm of breathing: normal breathing occurs at regular intervals. Irregular patterns may be indicative of brain injury or central nervous system damage or depression (particularly if the patient has reduced consciousness); or chest or abdominal injuries may be particularly painful and inhibiting of respiration (e.g. fractured ribs).

– Assess the depth of breathing: shallow breathing may not enable adequate gaseous exchange, possibly causing hypoxia and/or hypercarbia. Again, central nervous system depression or upper body injury may be factors. Excessively deep breathing may be due to the patient striving to take in more oxygen or expel carbon dioxide. Once more, the patient's emotional state may contribute.

– See whether or not the chest is moving evenly on both sides, and in both upper and lower areas (it should be!). It is often also helpful to place your hands on the lower ribcage – one hand on each side – to simultaneously feel chest movements (with due respect to patient dignity). Relatively less movement on one side or the other is suggestive of a blockage in one of the main bronchi on that side, or a considerable area of pulmonary consolidation, or a volume of air or fluid (of whatever kind) within the pleural cavity.

– If chest movement is only present on one side, check the position of the trachea: it should be centrally located (i.e. in the midline of the neck). Deviation towards one side or the other may be a sign of significant and even dangerous pulmonary disease (e.g. a large pleural effusion or tension pneumothorax (trachea is deviated away from the problem side), or lung collapse (trachea is deviated towards the problem side)). Such a deviation may be obvious from visual inspection but it can be helpful to use a finger to trace the trachea down the neck.

– Look for signs that breathing is effortful, such as flaring of the nostrils, intercostal recession (the tissue between the ribs is 'sucked in' during inspiration, particularly in the lower areas of the chest), use of accessory muscles of respiration (e.g. the scalene muscles in the neck; the tendons in the neck may stand out too), or so-called paradoxical breathing (instead of moving together, the chest and abdomen separately and alternately move in and out during respiration – so-called 'seesaw respirations'). The whole process of breathing may be difficult, but it may be that the patient finds it relatively more effortful to inspire (e.g. due to some degree of upper airway constriction) or to expire (e.g. in asthma).

- There may be tissues or a sputum pot in the vicinity of the patient. If so, it is worth having a look at any secretions, noting consistency, colour, quantity – and even the smell. Yellow or green, or thick/creamy, secretions are indicators of infection.

 Listen to the patient

- Normal conversation suggests that cerebral oxygenation is satisfactory at this point.
- Inability to complete a sentence (of ten words or more) without stopping to take a breath – or trying to talk but failing – are signs of severe respiratory compromise.
- Confused or inappropriate speech or incomprehensible sounds may be markers of reduced consciousness due to cerebral hypoxia.

 Listen to the breath sounds

Listen, firstly, by simply positioning yourself in front of the patient and listening. Normal breathing is sometimes barely audible without a stethoscope, but breathing in respiratory failure is often noisy and useful information can often be obtained even without auscultation.

- Abnormal breath sounds that may be heard in patients with respiratory disease include, for example, *rattling* sounds that may be indicative of secretions or fluid in the upper airways. If these sounds are heard, ask the patient to cough and expectorate, if possible, or consider using a Yankeur sucker to clear the oral cavity if the patient cannot expel this material.

- There may be the high-pitched sound of *stridor* (heard on inspiration), which is suggestive of a narrowing or partial obstruction of the upper airways. This is likely to be a very serious problem, and even life threatening, which should trigger an urgent call to (at the very least) the team with primary medical responsibility for the patient, and the outreach team or equivalent, if available.

- Also high-pitched, and with a whistling or hissing quality, is *wheeze*. This is the sound made by the movement of air through narrow airways (most often in the lower respiratory tract, and on expiration): e.g. with bronchoconstriction in asthma, or COPD, and sometimes in heart failure (cardiac asthma).

- It may even be possible to hear *crackles*, created by the movement of air through small airways when there are excessive secretions or fluid present (e.g. due to infection or pulmonary oedema). Generally, secretions cause what are called 'coarse crackles' and fluid gives rise to 'fine crackles', although the difference is not always clear cut – and, of course, it is quite possible to have infection and pulmonary oedema at the same time. The sound of coarse crackles can be altered or even eliminated by coughing or other means designed to mobilise secretions; while fine crackles (generally due to fluid) are not usually changed by these measures.

Rattling sounds, stridor and wheeze can often (but not always) be heard without a stethoscope, although crackles tend to be more difficult to hear. However, breath sounds will most easily be heard with a stethoscope, with the advantage that they can be more readily identified as coming from the right or left side of the chest, and from the upper, middle or lower lung zones. Auscultation (using a stethoscope) is a key part of any thorough examination of the respiratory system. It is easiest if the patient is sitting up and breathing reasonably, but not excessively deeply,

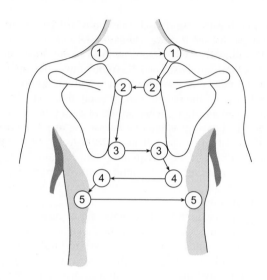

Fig. 5.4 Sequence for auscultation
From Cox C, Physical Assessment for Nurses, copyright 2004 with permission of Blackwell Publishing

in and out through an open mouth. It is important to listen to the chest in an ordered sequence (see Figure 5.4) in which the sounds at a particular level on one side of the chest are compared with those on the other side, checking whether breath sounds can be heard at all, whether the volume of sound is more or less than normal (compare with your own or a colleague's breath sounds to hear what is normal (hopefully)), and is similar on both sides.

Several different sorts of breath sounds can be heard in health:

1. The main sounds of breathing (called vesicular sounds) are soft and low pitched and can be heard over most of the lung fields, particularly away from the central area. They are sometimes said to sound a little like the rustling of dry leaves. The inspiratory phase is longer than the expiratory phase.
2. Louder, medium-pitch bronchovesicular sounds are heard over the bronchi either side of the sternum (breastbone) below the clavicles (collarbones), or between the scapulae (shoulder

blades) when listening to the back. The inspiratory and expiratory phases are about equal in length.

3. Louder still, higher pitch bronchial sounds can be heard from the large airways when listening over the manubrium (upper part of the sternum). Importantly, it is abnormal to hear bronchial sounds elsewhere in the chest; if these are heard in another location, it is usually because sounds of air movement in large airways are being transmitted through an area of consolidated tissue (e.g., with pneumonia). There is a pause between the sounds of inspiration and expiration; and the inspiratory phase is shorter than the expiratory phase.

Also, ask the patient to cough. This will help reveal whether the patient is able to obey commands (which will assist in the more detailed assessment of consciousness that will come later). It will give some information about the strength the patient can bring to an important function (a weak or absent cough is a marker of a more vulnerable patient, while pain in coughing should prompt consideration of the cause – and a possible need for analgesia) and it may yield sputum that can be examined (and, if appropriate, sent for laboratory analysis). In addition, a good cough is a very effective way of clearing airways.

 Feel – percussion

Percussion of the chest can help identify abnormalities in different parts of the lungs (see Chapter 3: Assessment Techniques). As in auscultation, an ordered sequence should be used, comparing, in turn, one side with the other, in the upper, mid and lower lung zones. Generally, percussion of the intercostal spaces (rather than the ribs) makes it easier to identify sounds heard related to the presence of air or different sorts of tissue underlying the area being percussed. A low-pitched, hollow (resonant) sound is expected from normal lungs (listen to your own chest to be sure what is normal), while a duller sound comes from consolidated tissue or the presence of fluid (e.g. pneumonia, oedema or pleural effusion). A more drum-like, hyper-resonant sound is heard when there is more air than usual (e.g. in a hyperinflated chest, as found in emphysema or severe asthma), or with a pneumothorax.

Measure – and record

Measure and record the respiratory rate, and the oxygen saturation using a pulse oximeter. The normal values for these parameters have been discussed above – remembering that oxygen saturation should always be considered with reference to any oxygen therapy administered.

OVERALL IMPRESSION OF THE PATIENT/NEXT STEPS/ DECIDING ON FIRST-LINE TREATMENT

If the patient is hypoxaemic/breathless, ask why, and where in the respiratory tract is the problem, and – most importantly – is this is a life-threatening illness requiring immediate expert assistance? If in doubt, always get advice. Consider:

- *Could the patient be better positioned?* Even if it is difficult, it is almost always worth sitting the patient up.
- *Is bronchoconstriction possible?* Give 2.5–5.0 mg nebulised salbutamol (driven by oxygen – not air – if the patient is already on 35% oxygen therapy).
- *Is there likely to be fluid, sputum, blood in the lungs or pleural cavity?* A chest x-ray will be useful in this case, and referral to a respiratory physiotherapist for expert input on clearing the alveoli. Pulmonary oedema may be due to acute heart failure, in which case a 12-lead ECG should be recorded and urgent expert help obtained.
- *Are there signs of a pneumothorax?* If so, seek help from a senior doctor. Again, a chest x-ray will be needed, and it may be that a chest drain is required (as may be the case if there is some kind of fluid in the pleural cavity).
- *Could pulmonary embolism be part of the problem?* Once more, chest x-ray is used to help differentiate the various diseases

that cause breathlessness, and a 12-lead ECG may reveal abnormalities associated with pulmonary embolism. A ventilation/perfusion (V/Q) scan or, more commonly, a computed tomographic pulmonary angiogram (CTPA) will be required for more definite diagnosis.

Key Points

Monitor the respiratory rate and work of breathing (i.e. the effort to breathe). A rising respiratory rate (e.g. ≥25 breaths/minute) or falling respiratory rate (e.g. ≤8 breaths/minute) indicate that the patient is deteriorating, so call the patient's medical team and the outreach team or equivalent (if available).

Give oxygen therapy to achieve the target oxygen saturations described above – and monitor the oxygen saturation, remembering that the more increasing concentrations of oxygen are required to reach these targets, the more the patient is at-risk of further deterioration.

SUMMARY

Breathing is the process by which the body takes in oxygen – the most important element for life. Difficulty in breathing is the single most common cause of hospitalisation: this may be due to disease of the respiratory tract itself or a complication of other illnesses such as disorders of the cardiovascular system. Patient assessment should always include, as a minimum, looking at, talking to and listening to the patient; looking at chest movement (e.g. rate and depth of movement) and whether or not the breathing is effortful; listening to breath sounds; and measuring respiratory rate. An abnormal respiratory rate – usually an increasing rate – is frequently one of the first signs of severe illness and should always be reported. It is critically important that the practitioner is clear about whether or not there is enough oxygen in the blood, by measuring oxygen saturation or checking an arterial blood gas (with consideration of whether the patient is just breathing air, or is requiring supplemental oxygen). Common causes of respiratory failure include infection, bronchoconstriction (e.g. asthma), fluid in the lungs or between the pleural membranes, pulmonary embolism or exacerbation of long-term diseases such as chronic obstructive pulmonary disease. Simple measures such as repositioning will often help the patient breathe more easily, and it is absolutely vital that adequate oxygen therapy is given when needed, remembering that a falling oxygen saturation and/or an increasing need for supplementary oxygen can be indicators of life-threatening deterioration.

CHAPTER 5: SCENARIOS

Scenario 5.1

A health care assistant asks you to see one of the patients on the ward: she has recorded his vital signs and reports that there is an abnormality, i.e. the pulse is fast. You know that the patient is a 32-year-old man admitted 4 days previously with traumatic fracture of the left lower leg (tibia and fibula) which occurred while he was playing football. He has had a surgical repair of the fracture (open reduction and internal fixation) and had seemed to be making a good recovery.

Q 1 What would you assess?

As you approach the patient, you see that he is slumped in the bed. When you ask 'how are you', he replies 'oh, my chest feels so tight' but seems to have difficulty getting the words out. You can hear a wheezing sound as the patient exhales. It can be seen that he is breathing fast and using accessory muscles of respiration.

Q 2 What do these first signs indicate?

Q 3 What should you do?

Q 4 What should you do next?

You find that that the patient has a respiratory rate of 34 breaths/minute and there is poor chest expansion. If auscultation is performed, quiet breath sounds can be heard throughout the chest with a high-pitched wheeze on expiration. The oxygen saturation is 91% (with the patient breathing oxygen at a flow rate of 15l/minute.

Q 5 *What do these data tell you?*

Q 6 *What else should be done?*

Answers to scenario 5.1

Q1 You would aim to obtain an initial impression of the patient, and then assess, each in turn, Airway–Breathing–Circulation–Disability–Everything else (A–B–C–D–E).

Q2 The fact that the patient can talk means that the airway is patent although there may be some partial obstruction. The fact that the patient is having difficulty completing a sentence is a sign of significant respiratory compromise: this is also indicated by the presence of audible wheeze and tachypnoea, and by the effort of breathing.

Q3 You have observed signs of severe respiratory failure, which requires calling for immediate expert help (a call to the cardiac arrest team may be the best way of getting help and is entirely appropriate in this situation). You may or may not know the exact nature of the patient's problem, but this is an emergency situation and he should be given high-concentration, high-flow oxygen (i.e. using a mask with non-rebreathe reservoir bag and maximum oxygen flow). You should help the patient to sit up and reassure him that you are taking action to manage his respiratory distress.

Q4 You can now obtain more information about the patient's clinical status, which will help to determine the severity of his illness and aid a proper diagnosis. Look closer at his chest movement, assessing (and counting) the respiratory rate, pattern, depth and symmetry, and measure oxygen saturation.

Q5 Essentially, you have further confirmation of the severity of the patient's illness. Hearing breath sounds throughout the chest reduces the likelihood that any particular area is completely obstructed or collapsed; rather, these sounds are indicative of bronchoconstriction (you could therefore ask for a nebuliser circuit to be set-up, with 5 mg salbutamol and 0.5 mg ipratropium bromide). An oxygen saturation of 91% while breathing high-flow oxygen is another sign of very severe illness (you would normally expect a patient like this to have 100% saturation when breathing oxygen). In fact, this is a feature of life-threatening compromise: such a patient needs to have an immediate review by an anaesthetist as tracheal intubation and mechanical ventilation may be required. It may also be useful to give oxygen through nasal cannulae (at 6 l/ minute if possible) in addition to that administered through the mask with non-rebreathe reservoir. This will necessitate a second source of oxygen, perhaps using a cylinder from the cardiac arrest trolley.

Q6 So far, you have focused on airway and breathing – which is as it should be – and you should have obtained expert help. However, it is still necessary to assess the circulation (the health care assistant first called you because she found the patient to be tachycardic) and to ensure, at the very least, that there is venous access: intravenous fluids and drugs are almost always needed in emergency situations. Blood samples should be taken (consider the possibility that chest infection may be a contributing factor here) and an arterial blood gas analysis done to help decide whether artificial ventilation might be required. The patient is tachypnoeic, which would normally reduce the pCO_2, so even a normal and especially an increasing pCO_2 is a significant adverse sign. (Even if you are not able to take blood yourself, ask a colleague to get the necessary equipment, bottles and forms for blood samples so that these are immediately available when help arrives.)

Wheeze and probable bronchoconstriction have been found in this case: common causes include acute asthma or an allergic reaction (and perhaps anaphylaxis), or so-called cardiac asthma (due to heart failure), or exacerbation of

COPD (e.g. emphysema). Bearing in mind the patient's age and known ability to usually undertake strenuous exercise, chronic heart disease or emphysema is very unlikely.

Summary

This patient has potentially life-threatening respiratory compromise. It is imperative to obtain immediate expert help, to position him so as to best enable his breathing, and to maximise the oxygen input. Nebulised salbutamol is a key treatment, and in this case it must be given using oxygen, with additional oxygen via nasal cannula as required. Continuous doses may be needed.

It is still essential to assess Circulation, Disability and Everything else. You must ensure that there is sufficient blood flow to transport oxygen around the body (measure heart rate and BP at the very least, and record a 12-lead ECG if possible) and make certain that there is adequate intravenous access. You then need to check consciousness and be vigilant to safeguard against any reduction in consciousness further compromising the airway. Assessment of Everything else must include exposing the abdomen and limbs (it should be remembered that the patient is actually in hospital with a broken leg) and checking for any signs or symptoms of new physical injury, inflammation, infection, inadequate perfusion, bleeding, etc. Review of the patient's charts and medical notes ought to reveal any underlying disease or other factors that might help diagnose the cause of this acute episode.

Scenario 5.2

A 72-year-old woman has been admitted to the ward following a stroke 5 days previously, which has left her with a mild but improving right-sided weakness, some dysarthria (disordered speech) and dysphagia (difficulty swallowing). She has also been diagnosed with a chest infection that was believed to be improving with antibiotic therapy. The patient is known to have chronic obstructive pulmonary disease (COPD) and to sometimes experience angina on exertion.

At morning handover, she is reported to have become confused and restless in the last 2 hours. The nurses found it difficult to record vital sign observations, but oxygen saturation was recorded as 81%, and therefore 50% oxygen therapy has been applied. A doctor has been called to see the patient but has yet to arrive.

Q 1 You are taking over the patient's care. How would you go about assessing her?

You see that the patient is partly sitting up, although leaning to one side. She does not answer when you speak to her, but does open her eyes when you touch her on the shoulder. You can see the chest moving – symmetrically, and the respiratory rate is 26 breaths/minute. The patient is receiving oxygen at 10 l/minute through a standard face mask, and the pulse oximeter shows an oxygen saturation of 88% (with a heart rate of 90 beats/minute).

Q 2 What is your initial impression and immediate actions?

The patient does try to cough when you ask, but it makes no difference to the rattling sound and she does not seem to clear anything from her airway.

Q 3 Is there anything else that might be done at this point?

Q 4 Should the oxygen flow be increased – or decreased?

Auscultation of the chest reveals breath sounds – and therefore air entry – in both lungs. There are coarse crackly sounds – and some expiratory wheeze – in the right upper zone, with reduced sounds of air entry in the right lower zone as compared with the left.

Q 5 What do these sounds suggest?

Assessment of the circulation informs you that the heart rate is 95 beats/minute – and the pulse is irregular (this has not been noted before). The BP is 127/67 mm Hg and the patient feels warm and sweaty. An arterial blood gas is taken by the doctor, with results as below:

pH	7.38	(normal range 7.35–7.45)
pCO$_2$	4.4 kPa	(normal range 4.6–6.1 kPa)
HCO$_3^-$	19.3 mmol/l	(normal range 22–26 mmol/l)
pO$_2$	7.53 kPa	(normal range 11.3–13.3 kPa)

Q 6 What does the blood gas tell you and what else should be done?

Answers to scenario 5.2

Q1 You would use the A–B–C–D–E framework.

Q2 You have not yet done a formal assessment of consciousness, but your first interaction with the patient might suggest that she is suffering a reduced level of consciousness – so you should talk to her again to check. It has been seen that she is leaning to one side: this may be no different from how she has been previously, but it is also possible that she may have had another episode of cerebral ischaemia (which might potentially compromise the airway). You have already noted that the chest is moving – so the airway must be at least partly open, but the rattling sound is indicative of some degree of obstruction, perhaps due to liquid in the upper airways. You should ask the patient to try and cough to clear her throat. An oxygen saturation of 88% is normal for at least some patients with severe COPD but is a very low value considering that the patient is receiving high-concentration oxygen, and is therefore indicative of severe respiratory failure. You should ensure that expert help is imminent; if not, it should be sought.

Q3 You should try to re-position the patient in a more upright posture. If you can see any material at the back of the mouth, it may be possible to remove it using a Yankeur sucker. If this manoeuvre is unsuccessful, placement of a nasopharyngeal airway would facilitate suction of the pharynx; in this case, when this was done, thick yellowy-green secretions were obtained and the patient's breathing seemed less laboured.

Q4 This issue is open to some debate. National guidelines suggest that patients with chronically raised carbon dioxide levels (e.g. with COPD – as in this case) can be managed with a saturation of 88–92%. Indeed, on occasion some of this group of patients suffer respiratory and neurological depression when their oxygen saturations are raised above what is normal for them. It is of concern that this particular patient appears to have a reduced level of consciousness, but at the same time she is breathing rapidly, which is not likely in respiratory depression. Furthermore, the patient has a severe acute problem compounding several chronic illnesses: therefore, it would be inadvisable to reduce the oxygen flow in what could easily become a life-threatening situation. It would be useful to find out the patient's normal saturation: should it turn out to be significantly higher than 88%, it would be reasonable to increase the oxygen – as it would be if she deteriorated even more. More definitively, an arterial blood gas would show whether the patient was at risk of respiratory acidaemia (i.e. if there is a high pCO_2 with a low pH).

Q5 The coarse crackly sounds are probably due to the presence of secretions. The reduced sounds may be caused by an area of local collapse or perhaps by an abnormal quantity of fluid or air, e.g. in a pleural effusion or pneumothorax. (A chest x-ray would be useful in due course.) It was already known that the patient had a respiratory infection, but it is now evident that this is worsening. The wheeze sound may be a symptom of bronchoconstriction so nebulised salbutamol is indicated, and you should consider humidifying the patient's oxygen to ease the clearance of secretions.

In addition, urgent assessment by a physiotherapist would be beneficial. You should aim to obtain a sample of sputum for microbiological analysis, and to arrange for blood cultures to be taken. It would also be advisable to seek guidance from a microbiologist about different antibiotic therapies. These last points are important, but it is also imperative to continue the patient assessment: you could ask a colleague to make the necessary calls, i.e. help is needed to manage this patient properly.

Q6 The pH is in the normal range, but all other values are abnormal, i.e. the pO_2 indicates hypoxaemia (so the oxygen flow rate should be increased). The pCO_2 is low (which, in itself, you would expect to increase the pH), and the HCO_3^- is also low (which, in itself, you would expect to reduce the pH). This is severe Type 1 respiratory failure, with a compensated metabolic acidosis, i.e. the patient is hyperventilating to eliminate CO_2 in order to compensate for the metabolic acidosis signified by the low HCO_3^-. It should be remembered that patients with COPD will usually have a high pCO_2: this patient is hyperventilating and there is a real danger that she will begin to tire. (The cause of the metabolic acidosis has yet to be identified, but it is likely that sepsis is playing at least some part. The patient has a history of angina – and an irregular pulse – so there is also a possibility of an acute cardiac event: a 12-lead ECG should be recorded to look for signs of ischaemia.)

Further assessment of perfusion is essential, as is establishment of venous access, and taking blood samples for analysis, followed by assessment of Disability – particularly as the patient has already suffered a stroke, then Everything else.

Summary

The patient has several severe acute and chronic problems, and it is essential to be sure that the fundamental functions of maintaining a clear airway, the taking in of oxygen and the expiration of carbon dioxide are achieved without being too distracted by other issues – while still remembering that some of these other issues also need to be addressed in a timely fashion. This illustrates the importance of using a systematic approach and being clear about the priorities of care.

The patient described here is at high risk of further deterioration. You will need help to assess and manage her properly, and also to develop a plan of care for the next few hours and days that is agreed by the ward team with the patient, taking advice from microbiology and perhaps radiology, with contributions from the physiotherapist and other allied health professionals (e.g. with regard to the patient's ability to safely take food or drink by mouth). It may be that the patient needs to move to a higher level of care, or, should she stay on the ward, that there should be a discussion about an appropriate ceiling of treatment for her.

Scenario 5.3

Review these three sets of arterial blood gases (from real cases: refer to Appendix 1 for guidance if needed) and decide:

Example 1

pH	7.31	(normal range 7.35–7.45)
pCO_2	6.9 kPa	(normal range 4.6–6.1 kPa)
HCO_3^-	25.7 mmol/l	(normal range 22–26 mmol/l)
pO_2	9.3 kPa	(normal range 11.3–13.3 kPa)
SpO_2	88%	

Example 2

pH	7.29	(normal range 7.35–7.45)
pCO_2	4.8 kPa	(normal range 4.6–6.1 kPa)
HCO_3^-*	17.1 mmol/l	(normal range 22–26 mmol/l)
pO_2	11.1 kPa	(normal range 11.3–13.3 kPa)
SpO_2	95%	

Example 3

pH	7.35	(normal range 7.35–7.45)
pCO_2	7.1 kPa	(normal range 4.6–6.1 kPa)
HCO_3^-	29.0 mmol/l	(normal range 22–26 mmol/l)
pO_2	9.1 kPa	(normal range 11.3–13.3 kPa)
SpO_2	92%	

Q 1 *Is there hypoxaemia (pO$_2$ < 8 kPa or arterial oxygen saturation (SaO$_2$) <90%)?*

Q 2 *What is the pH and, specifically, is there alkalaemia (pH > 7.45) or acidaemia (pH < 7.35)?*

Q 3 *What is the respiratory component (pCO$_2$) and, specifically, is there a respiratory acidosis (pCO$_2$ > 6.1 kPa) or respiratory alkalosis (pCO$_2$ < 4.6 kPa)?*

Q 4 *What is the metabolic component (bicarbonate (HCO$_3^-$)) and, specifically, is there a metabolic acidosis (HCO$_3^-$ < 22 mmol/l) or metabolic alkalosis (HCO$_3^-$ > 26 mmol/l)?*

Q 5 *If the HCO$_3^-$ or pCO$_2$ were abnormal, have they made the pH abnormal?*

Q 6 *What sort of patient might have arterial blood gas values like these?*

Answers to scenario 5.3

Example 1

Q1 The patient is hypoxaemic: the SpO$_2$ is <90% (even though the pO$_2$ is 9.3 kPa).

Q2 The pH is low, indicating that the blood is relatively acid (i.e. there is acidaemia).

Q3 The pCO$_2$ is high (hypercarbia), which causes acidosis (i.e. a respiratory acidosis due to respiratory failure).

Q4 The HCO$_3^-$ is within the normal range and is not contributing to the acidosis.

Q5 The pH is abnormally low (acid), due to the abnormally high pCO$_2$.

Q6 This is a case of respiratory acidosis – which is uncompensated (i.e. there has been no change in the HCO_3^- to counteract the excess of acid created by the high pCO_2). There is also hypoxaemia – and with the hypercarbia – this is characteristic of Type 2 respiratory failure.

Example 2

Q1 The patient is not hypoxaemic, although the pO_2 and SpO_2 values would be considered relatively low in a young, fit person. However, if the patient was receiving oxygen therapy when the blood gas was taken, it is likely that these values would be suboptimal if the oxygen was discontinued, indicating that there might be some underlying acute illness or chronic disease.

Q2 The pH is low, indicating that the blood is relatively acid (i.e. there is acidaemia).

Q3 The pCO_2 is within the normal range and is not contributing to the acidosis.

Q4 The HCO_3^- is low, indicating metabolic acidosis.

Q5 The pH is abnormally low (acid), due to the abnormally low HCO_3^-.

Q6 This is a case of metabolic acidosis – which is uncompensated (i.e. there has been no change in the pCO_2 is counteract the excess of metabolic acid). Metabolic acidosis has several causes: a systematic patient assessment is required to identify the problem. Common causes of metabolic acidosis include tissue hypoxia (most often due to poor perfusion) and renal failure, perhaps diabetic ketoacidosis or loss of bicarbonate, e.g. due to severe diarrhoea.

Example 3

Q1 The patient is not hypoxaemic by the standard definition, although the pO_2 and SpO_2 values are relatively low. Again, if the patient was receiving oxygen therapy when the blood gas was taken, these values would almost certainly be suboptimal if the oxygen was discontinued, indicating underlying illness or disease.

Q2 The pH is in the normal range (albeit at the lower end of the normal range).

Q3 The pCO_2 is high (hypercarbia), which causes acidosis – i.e. a respiratory acidosis due to respiratory failure, although the pH is normal.

Q4 The HCO_3^- is high, indicating metabolic alkalosis.

Q5 Both the pCO_2 and the HCO_3^- are abnormally high, but balance each other out to create a normal pH.

Q6 This is a case of a fully compensated respiratory acidosis, i.e. the high pCO_2 has been balanced by a high HCO_3^-. These values are typical of a patient with stable chronic obstructive pulmonary disease.

REFERENCES

British Thoracic Society Standards of Care Committee (2002) Non-invasive ventilation in acute respiratory failure. Thorax 57(3):192–211

British Thoracic Society (2004) BTS Guidelines for the Management of Community Acquired Pneumonia in Adults, 2004 Update. British Thoracic Society, London

British Thoracic Society (2006) The Burden of Lung Disease (2nd edn). A statistics report from the British Thoracic Society 2006. British Thoracic Society, London

McMorrow CN, Mythen MG (2006) Pulse oximetry. Current Opinion in Critical Care. 12(3):269–271

O'Driscoll BR, Howard LS, Davison AG, on behalf of the British Thoracic Society (2008) BTS guideline for emergency oxygen use in adult patients. Thorax 63(Suppl. VI):vi1–vi68

Oh TE (2003) Oxygen therapy. In: Oh's Intensive Care Manual (5th edn) (Eds Bersten AD, Soni N). Butterworth-Heinemann, Edinburgh

Royal College of Physicians, British Thoracic Society, Intensive Care Society (2008) Non-invasive ventilation in chronic obstructive pulmonary disease: management of acute type 2 respiratory failure. Royal College of Physicians, London

West JB (2004) Respiratory Physiology: The Essentials (7th edn). Lippincott Williams & Wilkins, Baltimore

A–B–**C**–D–E: Circulation (and Circulatory Failure)

6

INTRODUCTION

The heart and circulatory system transport blood around the body to deliver oxygen and nutrients to the tissues and collect excess carbon dioxide and other waste products for elimination. However, cardiovascular diseases are very common: about 5.6 million people in England have been diagnosed with some form of cardiovascular disease, and in the UK overall these diseases cause more than 208,000 deaths a year – 36% of all deaths (Scarborough et al, 2008). As well as chronic disease, many hospital patients suffer acute circulatory failure caused by such conditions as hypovolaemia, sepsis and myocardial infarction.

This chapter sets out a systematic approach to assessment of the cardiovascular system, ways common problems may be identified, and also first-line treatments such as fluid resuscitation. Basic cardiac monitoring and central venous pressure measurement and evaluation are described in supplementary sections at the end of the chapter.

LEARNING OBJECTIVES

By the end of this chapter you should be able to:

❑ Understand the role of each component of the circulatory system in transporting oxygen around the body
❑ Outline key aspects of fluid balance in health and illness
❑ Describe signs, symptoms and common causes of circulatory failure and shock
❑ Detail a systematic approach to rapid cardiovascular assessment
❑ Outline how the circulation can be monitored in a ward setting

❏ Discuss the indications for fluid resuscitation, and how this may be done
❏ Understand when expert help may be needed.

ANATOMY AND PHYSIOLOGY REFRESHER

The heart (Figure 6.1)

The heart is a cone shaped muscular pump –about 12 cm long, 9 cm wide, and 6 cm thick – sited between the lungs in the mediastinum. Two-thirds of its mass lie to the left of the midline. The heart contains four chambers: the atria (relatively thin-walled, low-pressure blood reservoirs and conduits) and ventricles (thick-walled, high-pressure blood pumps). The right atrium receives blood from the systemic circulation and channels it to the right ventricle for ejection into the pulmonary circulation. The

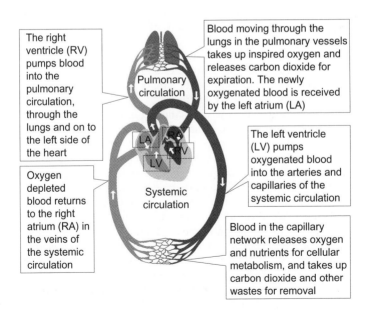

The right ventricle (RV) pumps blood into the pulmonary circulation, through the lungs and on to the left side of the heart

Oxygen depleted blood returns to the right atrium (RA) in the veins of the systemic circulation

Blood moving through the lungs in the pulmonary vessels takes up inspired oxygen and releases carbon dioxide for expiration. The newly oxygenated blood is received by the left atrium (LA)

The left ventricle (LV) pumps oxygenated blood into the arteries and capillaries of the systemic circulation

Blood in the capillary network releases oxygen and nutrients for cellular metabolism, and takes up carbon dioxide and other wastes for removal

Pulmonary circulation

Systemic circulation

LA   RA   RV   LV

Fig. 6.1 The flow of blood through the body

left atrium receives blood from the pulmonary circulation and channels it to the left ventricle for pumping into the aorta and systemic circulation.

The rate and force of cardiac contraction are regulated by the autonomic nervous system. Nervous stimulation is controlled by the medulla oblongata in the brain stem. Catecholamines (adrenaline and noradrenaline) secreted by the adrenal medulla increase sympathetic excitation, causing the heart to contract more quickly and with more force (the so-called 'fight or flight' mechanism). Other factors such as serum electrolyte levels (e.g. potassium and calcium), carbon dioxide and acid concentrations also influence cardiac function, as do body temperature, the patient's affective state (mood or emotion), gender and age. Most importantly, the heart requires a continuous supply of oxygen.

The circulatory system

The circulatory system has two main components: the systemic circulation and the pulmonary circulation. There are also several sub-systems, the most important of which is the coronary circulation.

The systemic circulation transports oxygenated blood from the left side of the heart to organs throughout the body and returns deoxygenated blood to the right side of the heart to be re-oxygenated in the pulmonary circulation. Vasomotor tone is vital in the control of the systemic circulation. It is able to maintain perfusion of vital organs in situations of relatively high and low blood volumes under a wide range of pressures, constricting and dilating arteries to vary the resistance to blood flow, channelling flow to particular regions of the body. Control is mediated centrally and peripherally. The autonomic nervous system is assisted by hormones such as adrenaline and noradrenaline and other vasoconstrictors, and by the endocrine system with antidiuretic hormone. Autoregulation occurs at a local level. Overall, there may be general effects of systemic vasoconstriction or vasodilation, but there are also likely to be variations in different body systems, particularly in illness, when blood flow to some organs may be reduced while perfusion of other areas is preserved or enhanced. Many drugs can influence vasomotor tone, so there are opportunities for pharmacological intervention.

Blood flow through the system is driven by the pumping action of the heart, moving from the high-pressure left ventricle (typically, pressure > 100 mmHg) to the low-pressure right atrium (pressure about 4 mmHg). Flow is governed by the size of the pressure gradient, with resistance determined by blood vessel length, and particularly by variations in blood vessel diameter and blood viscosity.

In comparison to the systemic circulation, the pulmonary circulation is a low-pressure, low-resistance and low-capacity system. This means that high volumes or high pressures in the pulmonary circulation are not easily absorbed and are therefore likely to cause complications such as pulmonary oedema (see below). The pulmonary circulation carries deoxygenated blood from the right side of the heart to the lungs for oxygenation and then takes oxygenated blood on to the left side of the heart for delivery throughout the body.

In the coronary circulation, the right and left coronary arteries come off the aorta at the coronary ostia. Usually, the left coronary artery and its offshoots supply the left atrium, left ventricle, intra-ventricular septum, anterior right ventricle and entire apex of the heart. The right coronary artery and its branches supply the right atrium, sinoatrial and atrioventricular nodes, right ventricle and posterior left ventricle. Five percent of cardiac output goes to the coronary circulation at rest, but increases in cardiac workload can require 25% of cardiac output to supply the heart muscle with oxygen. Most coronary perfusion occurs during the brief period after each ventricular contraction (i.e. during diastole); therefore, high heart rates – with necessarily shorter diastolic periods – tend to impair coronary perfusion.

Key Point

Getting oxygen to the tissues requires several components to be in place:

1. *The heart to pump an **adequate volume of blood.*** The performance of the pump can be determined by measuring the volume of blood ejected by the left ventricle into the systemic circulation with each contraction. This value may be represented by the ejection fraction (EF), i.e. the proportion of

ventricular blood volume ejected, which is normally at least 55%. The EF can be measured by echocardiography (cardiac ultrasound), which may be done at the bedside in many hospitals. More crudely, the pulse volume can be palpated by hand. The volume of blood pumped in one minute is termed the cardiac output.

2. *The blood needs to contain a* **sufficient concentration of haemoglobin** *(Hb) to which oxygen can attach.*

3. *The* **haemoglobin needs to be well saturated with oxygen** *(SaO_2).*
   Therefore, oxygen delivery is determined by volume of blood flow, haemoglobin, and oxygen saturation.

4. *In addition, blood must be pumped at an* **adequate pressure** *to perfuse vital organs.* If the heart pumps enough volume, the pressure generated is usually sufficient, but this is not always the case.

   Thinking about these four aspects of the circulation (blood flow, Hb, SaO_2, blood pressure) − and how well body organs are perfused and function − is a useful way to structure a review of the cardiovascular system.

BODY FLUID AND FLUID BALANCE (AFTER GUYTON AND HALL, 2006)

As the function of the cardiovascular system is to pump blood, and blood is mostly fluid (largely water), a working knowledge of basic principles of fluid balance is necessary for a proper understanding of the circulation. In fact, water makes up about 60% of total body mass, with some variation due to age, gender, race and individual body type (e.g. because muscle contains more water than fat).

The three fluid compartments (sometimes called fluid spaces) are separated by semi-permeable membranes through which water and a range of substances can pass, but other material cannot. The movement of fluid across these membranes is subject to various forces and restraints.

Fluid movement between fluid compartments

The pressure of blood in capillaries (hydrostatic pressure) tends to drive fluid out of the vascular compartment and into the interstitial compartment. At the same time, albumin and other

---

Box 6.1 Body fluid distribution in the three fluid compartments

Vascular compartment	3 l plasma		
Interstitial compartment	11 l interstitial fluid	Extracellular fluid	Total body water: 42 L
Intracellular compartment	28 l intracellular fluid	+ Intracellular fluid	=
Non-fluid mass	28 kg		
Total body mass	70 kg: weight of the so-called average man *(The average man today actually weighs 20% more than this. However, the proportions of fluid in the fluid compartments will be the same.)*		

---

proteins in the plasma act to counter outflow of fluid from the vascular compartment and even to draw fluid in. Proteins have more mass than water molecules and do not easily pass through the capillary membrane. The proteins in plasma effectively reduce the water content of the plasma (because they take up space that could otherwise be occupied by water) and create what is called colloid osmotic pressure, meaning that water in a more dilute fluid (e.g. in the interstitial compartment) will tend to move into the vascular compartment so as to equilibrate water concentrations in the two adjacent compartments (Box 6.1).

The effects of these opposing and variable forces can be seen, for example, when there is elevated hydrostatic pressure in the pulmonary circulation (e.g. due to heart failure), which leads to movement of fluid into the pulmonary interstitial compartment and then the alveoli of the lung, causing pulmonary oedema. This fluid flux occurs with much lower hydrostatic pressures when there are also reduced plasma protein levels (i.e. when colloid osmotic pressure is relatively low).

The permeability of membranes between fluid compartments is another variable. Processes of systemic inflammation and infection can damage vascular endothelium, resulting in increased 'capillary leak' of fluid from the circulation. There is normally relatively little plasma protein in the interstitial compartment, but if the membrane becomes more permeable, there may also be a significant shift of protein into the interstitial compartment. This will decrease the colloid osmotic pressure of the vascular compartment – further reducing the retention and inflow of fluid into the circulation – and promote more fluid accumulation in the interstitial compartment. If this process continues, hypovolaemia – i.e. reduced blood volume – will occur. It is entirely appropriate to treat hypovolaemia with administration of intravenous fluids in order to maintain an adequate blood pressure, but these fluids will also tend to leak out of the vascular compartment in due course. The phenomenon of systemic capillary leak can result in a situation where total body water is much higher than normal – because interstitial and eventually intracellular fluid volumes are increased – and the patient is grossly oedematous, but also hypovolaemic and hypotensive. These are difficult patients to manage. They require a balance of sufficient intravenous fluid to maintain blood pressure and perfusion of vital organs, but also consideration of how excessive accumulations of fluid in other areas can be minimized – because such accumulations tend to hamper the free movement of oxygen and nutrients to the cells as well as making tissue more fragile (e.g. causing wound dehiscence).

Electrolytes in body fluids

Body fluids contain material such as blood cells (in the vascular compartment, but not normally in the other compartments, lipids, and proteins (primarily in the vascular and intracellular compartments but less in the interstitial compartment). There are also many electrolytes and other substances dissolved in body fluids. For example, there are large quantities of sodium and chloride in extracellular fluid, but not much potassium or phosphate; while there is normally little sodium or chloride in cells, but high levels of potassium and phosphate. These differences in electrolyte concentration between intracellular and extracellular compartments are maintained because cell membranes have particular qualities of selective permeability – favouring admission of potassium over sodium – and mechanisms of active transportation that moves any sodium that enters the cell right out again while actively bringing potassium in. The capillary membranes between the vascular and interstitial compartment do not have these properties so electrolyte levels in the vascular and interstitial compartments are more or less the same. The concentrations of different substances in body fluids can be measured in the laboratory (e.g. using a blood sample to determine plasma levels of sodium, potassium, glucose or creatinine); and are also reflected in the osmolarity of the fluid.

Osmolarity is an indicator of the quantity of material dissolved in a solution – and also of the relative water content of the fluid. If some substance is dissolved in a fluid, the concentration of water is reduced – shown by a higher measured osmolarity. The lower the measured osmolarity, the more dilute the fluid. When there are two fluids with different concentrations of water separated by a semi-permeable membrane, water will tend to move across the membrane from the relatively dilute fluid to the fluid with a lower water concentration. This principle is illustrated in the practice of sprinkling slugs with salt in order to kill them. Slugs have high water content and a semi-permeable, slimy skin. Salt placed on the slug's skin creates a very concentrated solution (with high osmolarity), drawing water out of the slug's body and dehydrating it. Similarly, in the human body, increased sodium concentrations in extracellular fluid (hypernatraemia) will tend to draw water out of cells. Lower levels of extracellular sodium (hyponatraemia), and therefore reduced extracellular osmolarity, may lead to water shifting into cells where the osmolarity is maintained by potassium, phosphate etc. Rapid changes in extracellular sodium can cause large fluid shifts, sometimes resulting in such life-threatening conditions as cerebral oedema.

Fluid balance

As a general rule, there needs to be an average urine output of *at the very least* 0.5 ml per kg of body weight per hour if body waste products are to be eliminated through the kidneys. This equates to > 1 l of urine per day for an average size man. Water in faeces and insensible losses through the skin and lungs usually account for at least another litre of output. In this case, there will

Table 6.1 Typical daily fluid balance for a healthy adult

Input (ml)		Output (ml)	
Water as liquid	1200	Urine	1500
Water in food	1000	Faeces	100
Water from metabolism	300	Insensible losses	
		– from skin	450
		– from lungs	450
		(sweat not included, but may be < 8 l!).	
Total input	2500	Total output	2500

need to be a minimum of 2 l water input to ensure fluid balance; or, as a rough rule of thumb, water requirements in health can be calculated as about 25–35 ml/kg of bodyweight per day, or < 1.5 ml/kg of bodyweight per hour. It is worth remembering that there are significant quantities of water in foods, and that body metabolism produces water too; so the input does not all have to be liquid (see Table 6.1).

It is also worth remembering that a lot of fluid intake is not measurable in the ward setting (i.e. the water in food and from metabolism – which added together might easily make up half of daily water requirements – is difficult to estimate). Insensible losses are not measurable either. Therefore, although accurate charting of those fluid inputs and outputs that are measurable is an essential part of monitoring the acutely ill patient, physical assessment and some thought about the likely nature of immeasurable inputs and outputs are important too. Daily weighing of patients can also reveal increases and decreases in total body water.

Fluid balance is disturbed in illness – sometimes with an overall excess of body water, or an accumulation of fluid in one area and deficit in another. For example, although total body water may not change, there is a tendency for fluid to be lost from the cardiovascular compartment in illness due to such factors as increased capillary permeability and the reduction in plasma osmotic pressure associated with hypoalbuminaemia. In acute illness, the imbalance is most often hypovolaemia and/or general dehydration. The unwell patient tends to have reduced fluid intake while fluid losses are often larger than normal because of, for instance, increased respirations, sweating due to fever, diarrhoea and vomiting, trauma or surgery (particularly with drains or stoma formation), etc.

Compensatory physiological mechanisms are activated in cases of fluid deficit which further alter fluid and electrolyte distribution. These mechanisms are part of a larger set of processes – sometimes termed the stress response – triggered by acute physical injury of one kind or another (including surgery). The hormones angiotensin and vasopressin (antidiuretic hormone) cause systemic vasoconstriction and increase blood pressure. Angiotensin and vasopressin also – with aldosterone – act on the kidneys to retain the sodium and water normally excreted in urine. Potassium excretion may be increased. Elevated sodium levels work to enhance blood volume by drawing in fluid from the intracellular compartment.

SIGNS AND SYMPTOMS OF DEHYDRATION
Rapid fluid losses are usually signalled by changes in vital signs (see 'Signs and Symptoms of Circulatory Failure' below). Slower or smaller – but significant – fluid deficits may not be so obvious. Thirst, a dry mouth, difficulty swallowing and reduced skin elasticity may be found. Dehydration may be revealed by a raised plasma sodium concentration – and also elevated levels of albumin and haemoglobin/haematocrit. (Haematocrit is a measure of the percentage of blood volume taken up by red blood cells. This value is increased when the plasma volume is reduced.) Note that there may not necessarily be an increase in the absolute quantities of these substances, but rather the relative concentrations are elevated as water is lost from body fluid.

Deciding on replacement fluids (Low and Milne, 2007; Vincent and Weil, 2006)
It is almost always preferable for patients to take fluids by mouth, or, failing that, by enteral tube (nasogastric/gastrostomy/jejunostomy tube). However, in gastrointestinal failure or when rapid fluid infusions are required, intravenous fluids are needed. There is no fluid that is appropriate for all situations, or not on a

continuous basis. Choice of fluid therapy should be guided by an assessment of which body fluid compartments are particularly depleted, the size of the fluid deficit, some consideration of electrolyte balance, and perhaps whether or not the membranes surrounding fluid compartments are likely to be more permeable than normal. The patient history, physical examination, blood results and scrutiny of fluid charts can all contribute to informed decision making.

There is a wide range of fluids available for intravenous administration, commonly categorised in three main groups (see Table 6.2). These fluids vary in what is dissolved in them; osmolarity (i.e. how dilute or concentrated they are); and whether or not they contain any large-size material. Price may also be a factor: crystalloid fluids are relatively inexpensive – less than £1.00 per litre – whereas colloids can cost at least ten times more.

- Crystalloids are solutions of low-mass salt and/or sugar molecules. These molecules are small enough to pass freely through

Table 6.2 Characteristics of commonly used intravenous fluids

	Sodium content (mmol/l)	Osmolarity (mOsm/l)	Molecular weight (da)
Crystalloids			
5% glucose	0	279	
Compound sodium lactate (Hartmann's)	131	280	
Sodium chloride 0.9% ('normal saline')	154	308	58
Colloids			
Gelatine (e.g. succinylated gelatine ('Gelofusine'®))	154	274	30,000
Etherified starch (e.g. 6% hydroxyethyl starch ('Voluven'®))	154	308	130,000
Plasma	134–146	275–295	69,000
Albumin		300	

Note: There is some variation in the composition of colloids made by different manufacturers, and in the normal ranges of blood results given by different laboratories.

the semi-permeable membranes between fluid compartments (e.g. the molecular weight of sodium chloride 0.9% – so-called 'normal saline' – is just 58 daltons). Other crystalloids include Hartmann's solution and 5% glucose.

- Synthetic colloids contain salt but also much higher mass, larger molecules, usually manufactured from gelatine or corn starch. These molecules move less easily through semi-permeable membranes: typical gelatine-based fluids have a mean molecular weight of 30,000 daltons, while etherified starch averages 130,000 daltons.
- Blood and blood products include whole blood, packed red blood cells, fresh frozen plasma, and human albumin solutions, containing a variety of higher mass, larger size material (e.g. the molecular weight of albumin is 69,000 daltons).

It can be seen from the table that most intravenous fluids contain sodium. In fact, sodium chloride 0.9% ('normal saline') and the two colloids in the table contain significantly more sodium than the body's own plasma: 'normal saline' is not normal at all! As discussed above, sodium in the body is mostly found in the extracellular compartments. This means that when intra-venous fluids containing sodium are administered, they will tend to spread through the vascular compartment and then into the interstitial compartment, but will not move so readily into the intracellular compartment. Large volumes of high-sodium solu-tions may even increase extracellular sodium to the point where intracellular water is drawn out of the cells – increasing extracel-lular fluid volume, but with the potential to shrink the cells. Normal saline, gelatine and etherified starch-based fluids also contain considerable amounts of chloride (110–154 mmol/l). Large volumes of these fluids may cause hyperchloraemia, which can increase acid levels in the body.

Colloids – especially starch-based colloids – contain molecules that are less likely to move rapidly though capillary membranes (starches may even have a sealant effect that reduces capillary permeability). These fluids are therefore retained in the vascular compartment longer than crystalloids, so smaller volumes are required if it is simply vascular fluid loss that is being treated (remembering that it may be replacement blood that is needed most: see below). In addition, fluids with higher molecular weight molecules may increase the total colloid osmotic pressure of the vascular compartment, drawing in fluid from the interstitial compartment and enhancing expansion of blood volume. However, some colloids have been reported to cause anaphylaxis, clotting disorders, and renal dysfunction.

Compound sodium lactate (Hartmann's) solution contains less sodium and chloride than normal saline, as well as quantities of potassium and calcium similar to those found in plasma. It is recommended as a first-line treatment in trauma, although it will tend to move quite quickly from the vascular compartment and into the interstitial compartment. Indeed, as sodium and osmolarity levels in sodium lactate solution are lower than normal extracellular fluid, it may be that some of the water content will be taken up by the intracellular compartment too. This could be useful if cells are dehydrated, but not if they are fluid overloaded. Therefore, sodium lactate solution is not recommended for patients with significant oedema, particularly cerebral oedema.

By definition, 5% glucose contains just water and 50 g glucose per litre. It will quickly be distributed throughout all three body fluid compartments so that it is a good treatment for dehydration, but not useful if the patient is oedamatous. Five per cent glucose has no value in hypovolaemia: for every litre given to the average-size man, less than 100 ml will be retained in the vascular compartment for any significant time.

Deciding on replacement fluids – summary

- Compound sodium lactate, sodium chloride 0.9%, and colloids may all be used to increase circulating blood volume (as may transfusion of blood or blood products). The colloids – particularly starch-based colloids – are likely to stay longest in the vascular compartment, especially if there is increased capillary leakage (e.g. in systemic infection and inflammation; or with hypoalbuminaemia: look for signs of systemic oedema). Therefore, smaller volumes of colloid may be used to restore blood volume. However, possible side-effects of colloids place some limits on how much should be given (e.g. no more than 3.5 l etherified starch per day to a 70 kg man), particularly if the patient has a clotting disorder. Colloids are also relatively expensive.

- If serum sodium levels are already high, sodium chloride 0.9% will tend to exacerbate this abnormality, and over time may lead to increased total body water (and oedema). Even if serum sodium levels are normal, it should be noted that the UK Food Standards Agency recommends that adults in everyday life have no more than 2.5 g sodium a day: 1 l sodium chloride 0.9% contains 9 g.
- For different reasons, compound sodium lactate solution and 5% glucose are likely to perpetuate problems of oedema. However, both fluids are useful for treatment of dehydration.
- Excess (metabolic) acid in the body may be increased by excessive chloride (especially in sodium chloride 0.9%).

Key Point

As a general rule, think carefully before giving any more than, say, half the patient's daily fluid requirement in just one form of intravenous fluid, and avoid giving more than 1 l sodium chloride 0.9% a day – unless the patient is known to be sodium or chloride depleted. Overall, compound sodium lactate or something similar is generally the most appropriate crystalloid fluid; although new, more balanced crystalloid and colloid solutions will become available in the near future: these solutions have electrolyte content much more like that of plasma. If just simple solutions of sodium chloride and glucose are used, the patient will probably also need potassium supplementation in some form or other.

ISSUES TO CONSIDER WHEN ASSESSING THE PATIENT

Is blood volume and flow adequate?

Blood flow or cardiac output can actually be measured in some settings, although not often on general wards. It is important to understand the four main factors that influence cardiac output:

1. The volume of blood in the heart before it contracts – basically, venous return – is the key influence on cardiac preload: that is, the force stretching cardiac muscle fibres before they contract. This is important because stretching the cardiac muscles – unless they are overstretched – increases the force of contraction:
   - if overall blood volume is low, reduced venous return will tend to decrease the preload and lower cardiac output;
   - but excessive blood volume can overload the heart and reduce its ability to function effectively.

   Preload is also affected by vascular tone (the dilation or constriction of blood vessels), cardiac muscle mass and other factors.

2. The intrinsic strength of cardiac muscle contraction. The strength of contraction is reduced by coronary heart disease and such problems as electrolyte imbalances and cardiac dysrhythmias (e.g. atrial fibrillation) that prevent coordinated contraction of the heart.

3. The tone of the arterial circulation into which the heart pumps is the main component of what is sometimes called afterload – that is, the resistance to the ejection of blood from the heart presented by the state of the vascular system:
   - if the arteries are relatively constricted, resistance to blood flow is increased and cardiac output may decrease,
   - but if the arteries are dilated, although it is easy for the heart to pump blood and cardiac output may be high, pressure in the system (i.e. blood pressure) can fall.

4. The heart rate:
   - very fast heart rates (e.g. over 150/minute) are so rapid that the heart chambers are not likely to properly fill with blood before contraction, so output will be reduced,
   - however, very slow heart rates (e.g. under 40/minute) may also mean that insufficient blood is pumped.

Key Point

Abnormally fast heart rates (tachycardias) are generally defined as rates > 100 beats/minute, and slow heart rates (bradycardias) as < 60 beats/minute. If the measured heart rate is outside the range 60–100 beats/minute, there should be some consideration of whether or not this is a sign of a significant problem, remembering that there may be cardiac and non-cardiac causes (e.g. respiratory distress, or anxiety). Blood flow and perfusion are not usually greatly affected until the heart rate is somewhat higher than 100 or lower than 60 beats/minute.

Is the haemoglobin concentration sufficient?

The haemoglobin concentration can be obtained from measurement of the full blood count. Normal ranges are about 11.5–15.5 g/dl (women) and 13.5–17.5 g/dl (men).

If we consider the equation *oxygen delivery = blood flow* $\times$ *Hb* $\times$ *SaO*$_2$, it can be seen that if the Hb falls from, say, 14.0 g/dl to 7.0 g/dl, the amount of oxygen delivered is halved unless the cardiac output and/or oxygen saturation are increased. If the oxygen saturation is 90%, increasing it to the maximum possible level will improve oxygen delivery, but only by a relatively small amount (approximately 11%). Rather, to restore oxygen delivery to its previous level, there will have to be a large increase in blood flow – and therefore a large increase in cardiac work. This may be a problem for a diseased heart. Red blood cell transfusion to increase Hb concentration may be considered as an option, but this also has its hazards (because even cross-matched blood is 'foreign tissue' to the patient). Current practice is generally to maintain Hb levels at no less than 7.0–9.0 g/dl, with transfusion reserved for when the Hb falls below this range (Hébert et al, 2007). However, certain high-risk patients (e.g. with acute cardiac disease, acute bleeding, or in the early stages of septic shock) should be maintained at a higher minimum level of Hb – i.e. at least 8.0 to 10.0 g/dl (Hébert et al, 2007).

Is the haemoglobin well saturated?

Ensuring that the blood is well saturated with oxygen depends primarily on effective management of airway and breathing – with oxygen therapy as required (see Chapter 5).

Is the blood pressure adequate?

What is normal blood pressure?

Mean BP is 134/73 mmHg for men and 128/71 mmHg for women in England (Information Centre, 2006). BP need not increase with age, but it usually does in the populations of developed countries: for people 75 years or over, mean systolic BP is 141 mmHg for men and 144 mmHg for women (Information Centre, 2006).

It should be noted that the different components of blood pressure measurements can provide information about different aspects of cardiovascular performance:

- Systolic BP is essentially generated by the strength of cardiac contraction and the volume of blood pumped by that contraction, so low systolic pressure can be treated by fluid therapy or drugs that increase the force of contraction.
- Diastolic BP is related to arterial tone. Constricted vessels increase diastolic pressure and vasodilation lowers diastolic pressure. Drugs that vasodilate (e.g. glyceryl trinitrate) or vasoconstrict (e.g. adrenaline) can be used when appropriate.

Hypertension

Hypertension increases the risk of myocardial infarction and stroke. Hypertension is defined as a persistent systolic BP ≥ 140 or diastolic BP ≥ 90 mmHg (NICE, 2006). Persistent BP of ≥ 160/100 mmHg often needs drug treatment, while ≥ 180/110 mmHg requires immediate referral to a specialist (NICE, 2006). The NICE guidance is aimed at primary care, not acute hospital settings, but these figures can be used as indicators of problem levels.

Hypotension

As a general rule, a systolic BP < 90 mmHg or a diastolic BP of < 60 mmHg may be a sign of a significant problem and should prompt proper assessment of the patient's condition. A minority of patients normally have blood pressures at 90/60 mmHg or even lower, but these are usually either exceptionally fit individuals or people with long-term conditions (e.g. chronic heart failure, liver disease, some endocrine disorder). Note that if the patient's usual systolic BP is, say, 150 mmHg, then a sudden decrease to 105 mmHg is again probably indicative of a significant deterioration: i.e. a fall of > 40 mmHg from the patient's normal BP requires review.

How well are the body organs functioning?

Reduced blood flow and/or BP affects all body organs to a greater or lesser extent. Therefore, deterioration in organ function is often an indication of circulatory failure. For example:

- *The kidneys* To control electrolyte levels and eliminate waste products (e.g. urea, creatinine), an average person needs to produce at least 0.5 ml of urine per hour for every kg of bodyweight. Less than this indicates that the patient is at risk of developing renal failure. According to the Information Centre (2006), average bodyweight for men is 83.2 kg and 70.3 kg for women. Therefore, an average man should produce a minimum of about 42 ml urine/hour (~1000 ml/day), and an average woman at least 35 ml/hour (~840 ml/day). Acute renal failure is indicated by rising serum creatinine and falling urine output:
  - creatinine increased by 50% and/or urine output < 0.5 ml/ kg bodyweight/hour for ≥ 6 hours are signs that the patient is at risk of acute renal failure,
  - creatinine that has doubled and/or urine output < 0.5 ml/ kg/hour for ≥ 12 hours suggests that the patient has sustained kidney injury,
  - creatinine that has tripled (or is > 350 µmol/l) and/or urine output < 0.3 ml/kg/hour for ≥ 24 hours indicates actual acute renal failure (Bellomo et al, 2004).

Key Point

Note that baseline creatinine levels vary considerably with age, gender and race (e.g. from 71–133 µmol/l). For instance, a young black man would generally be expected to have a significantly higher creatinine than an elderly white woman (Bellomo et al, 2004).

Many factors affect renal function and urine output, but a very common cause of low urine output in hospital patients is inadequate blood flow or BP.

- *The brain* Drowsiness or confusion may have a number of causes, but low blood flow or BP should always be considered as a possibility (see Chapter 7, D–Disability).
- *Gastrointestinal tract* The absence of bowel sounds (normally generated by movement of the intestines) may be an indication of significantly reduced intestinal activity (ileus). Again, there may be a variety of reasons for this abnormality, but reduced blood flow to the bowel is one of the main causes.

SIGNS AND SYMPTOMS OF CIRCULATORY FAILURE

Haemorrhage

Consider Table 6.3, showing typical vital signs of patients with different volumes of blood loss. It can be seen that even when a large volume such as < 1500 mL of blood is lost (so-called 'Class II haemorrhage'), there are changes (increases) in heart rate and in respiratory rate, but systolic BP is generally maintained – by compensatory peripheral vasoconstriction (indicated by cooling of the hands and feet and an *increase* in diastolic BP). Marked hypotension, reduced urine output and depressed consciousness are often relatively late signs.

Table 6.3 American College of Surgeons Advanced Trauma Life Support classification of haemorrhage (values estimated for 70 kg male). Reproduced from *ATLS Student Course Manual* Eighth Edition 2008, American College of Surgeons, with permission

Severity of haemorrhage	Class I	Class II	Class III	Class IV
Blood loss (ml)	<750	750–1500	1500–2000	>2000
Heart rate (min^{-1})	<100	>100–120	>120–140	>140
Systolic BP (mmHg)	Normal	Normal	Decreased	Decreased
Respiratory rate (min^{-1})	14–20	20–30	30–40	>35
Urine output (ml/hour)	>30	20–30	5–15	Negligible
Mental status	Slightly anxious	Mildly anxious	Anxious, confused	Lethargic, confused

Sepsis

Signs of circulatory failure are among the key indicators of developing sepsis. The International Sepsis Definitions Conference group suggests that sepsis can be diagnosed when there is a confirmed or suspected infection and also some of a variety of indicators, including (Levy et al, 2003):

- core temperature above 38.3 °C/below 36 °C
- heart rate above 90/min
- respiratory rate above 30/min
- systolic BP below 90 mmHg or a systolic BP decrease > 40 mmHg
- altered mental state
- reduced urine output, i.e. < 0.5 ml urine/kg/hour for at least 2 hours
- ileus (absent bowel sounds), or
- abnormal blood tests:
  - *inflammatory markers:* white blood cell count > 12,000/μl– < 4,000/μl or plasma C-reactive protein increase (> 2 SD above the normal value)
  - creatinine increase ≥ 43 μmol/l
  - abnormal clotting: INR (international normalised ratio) > 1.5; aPTT (activated partial thromboplastin time) > 60 s
  - platelet count < 100,000/μl
  - total bilirubin > 70 mmol/l
  - lactate > 3 mmol/l.

Myocardial infarction

Circulatory failure can give rise to relatively subjective and non-specific signs and symptoms. For example, the warning signs of myocardial infarction (death of cardiac muscle tissue) may include (Thygesen et al, 2007):

- discomfort – not necessarily pain – (e.g. a feeling of heaviness or tightness; or a persistent dull ache in the central chest area) or crushing pain; sometimes including discomfort in one or both arms or in the back, neck, jaw or stomach
- shortness of breath
- sweating, nausea, light-headedness.

Myocardial infarction sometimes occurs with few obvious or no symptoms at all! But if the patient looks/feels unwell, patient assessment to check systemic perfusion and organ function is essential, together with recording and review of a 12-lead ECG if a cardiac problem is possible. Again, adverse signs such as hypotension, reduced consciousness, and oliguria are indicators of impending or actual organ failure.

CARDIOVASCULAR ASSESSMENT

The minimum requirement is to:

- **look** at – and talk to – the patient and
- **listen** to the response;
- **feel** the pulse (rate, rhythm, volume) – checking peripheral temperature at the same time;
- **measure** capillary refill, pulse rate and blood pressure (and urine output if possible).

On first approach, introduce yourself and say what you plan to do (i.e. perform an assessment). Ask 'how are you?'

 Look at the patient

- *What is his general appearance? Are there any immediately obvious abnormalities?*
  At any point in the examination, if it is evident that the patient is acutely unwell, consider the need for urgent expert help.
- *Is the patient pale or dusky, flushed, grey, or blue (all possible indicators of inadequate circulation) or sweaty?*
  Make a point of looking at the lips (and tongue if possible), and the hands and fingers too. Blue tinting (cyanosis) of the extremities is associated with reduced peripheral perfusion. This may be significant but not life-threatening. Blue lips and tongue (central cyanosis) indicate a serious respiratory or cardiovascular problem and oxygen therapy should be started if not already in place.

A dry mouth – and dry, furrowed or swollen tongue – may be signs of dehydration.

- *Are there wounds, rashes or mottling (patchy discoloration) to be seen?*

 Listen to the patient responses

 Feel

- *Palpate the radial pulse in the wrist: consider the rate, rhythm and volume.*
  If bradycardic or tachycardic, and especially if irregular or low volume, check the carotid pulse too (e.g. in the grooves either side of the larynx (Adam's apple) – but not both carotid pulses at the same time). It can be useful to check and compare pulses on both sides of the body. New abnormalities in the pulse require further investigation (e.g. a 12-lead ECG) and, generally, blood tests if not recently done. These can be requested while the physical examination continues.
  – Heart rates > 150 beats/minute or < 40 beats/minute are not likely to generate adequate cardiac output for a sustained period: seek prompt expert help in these cases.
  – Irregular rhythms have the potential to become more irregular – and life-threatening.
  – Difficult-to-palpate pulses are signs of low cardiac output. A strong, large volume, 'bounding' pulse should also be noted – a bounding pulse (usually with warm hands) may indicate sepsis.
- *Feel both of the patient's hands: are they warm or cold?*
  Warm, perhaps abnormally warm, hands suggest vasodilation. If they are cold, it suggests poor perfusion/vasoconstriction.
- *What is the elasticity of the skin like (i.e. skin turgor)?*

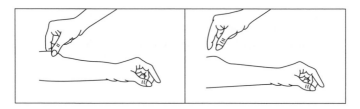

Fig. 6.2 Assessing skin turgor

Gently pinch a fold of skin on the arm (or back of the hand) and then release it. A skin fold that does not return to its usual state more or less immediately indicates dehydration (see Figure 6.2).

- *Feel both feet and ankles. Again, are they warm or cold?*
  If they are warm (or abnormally warm), it suggests vasodilation; if cold, poor perfusion. Also look for any swelling: ankle oedema may be indicative of chronic heart, kidney or liver disease; calf swelling a consequence of deep vein thrombosis. If the feet are cold, what about the ankles and calves? If most or all of the legs are cold, perfusion of the limbs and probably some vital organs is likely to be severely impaired.
  A study of 100 patients with shock showed that the temperature of the toes correlates well with cardiac output. That is, cold feet indicate low output, while warm toes are associated with an adequate – or increased – output (Joly and Weil, 1969). Blood pressure did not correlate well with output. What is more, toe temperature was also found to be a good predictor of outcome in these patients (Joly and Weil, 1969).

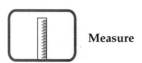 **Measure**

- *Measure the capillary refill time.*
  Press on a fingernail for 5 seconds so that it blanches (turns white), then release the pressure and determine how long

it takes the colour to return (usually no more than 2–3 seconds).

- – Capillary refill time > 3 seconds (particularly if there are other adverse signs – e.g. increased heart rate, increased respirations) indicates poor peripheral perfusion and therefore some degree of circulatory failure.
- – A brisk (fast) capillary refill might seem to be a good thing, but actually can be a sign of excessive vasodilation (e.g. in sepsis or anaphylaxis – or excessive vasodilatory medications, or epidural analgesia). The BP should be checked to ensure that it has not too low.

  Note: The finger pressed to check capillary refill should be more-or-less level with the patient's heart.

- *Measure and record the pulse rate, and the blood pressure.*

  Use a cuff that is empty of air before the procedure, fitted snugly around the arm and centred over the brachial artery. Too large a cuff will artificially lower the values recorded, while too small a cuff will give higher values than the patient's actual BP. It is recommended that the BP cuff bladder length is 80% of arm circumference, and the cuff width at least 40% of arm circumference (Pickering et al, 2005).

  - – Systolic BP < 90 mmHg, diastolic BP < 60 mmHg, or a fall of > 40 mmHg from the patient's normal BP are inadequate for most patients – or reflect some chronic disease process that also places the patient at risk.
  - – Remember that the systolic BP is essentially a function of the volume of venous return and the strength of cardiac contraction, while the diastolic BP is related to arterial tone.

Key Point

While checking the patient's hands, wrists and upper arms, make a point of noting the presence and appearance of any intravenous cannulae at these sites. There may of course be cannulae at other locations — and these should be noted – but the arms are the most commonly used sites.

- *Measure the urine output (if possible).*
  Urine output < 0.5 ml urine/kg/hour for 2 or more hours is generally considered abnormal and should be further investigated (e.g. check that the catheter is patent and draining freely, if there is one; check the patient's blood results – particularly, urea, creatinine, potassium – and consider sending a new blood sample for analysis if there appears to be a new problem).

 Look further

- Complete the examination by checking the abdomen and lower limbs if not already viewed, and rolling the patient on to one side to see the back: look for signs of fluid loss (e.g. blood, faeces), any drains, or areas of swelling/distension. Remember that it is possible for there to be very large volumes of internal fluid loss from the circulation following trauma or surgery or in conditions causing systemic inflammation (e.g. sepsis, pancreatitis). This may be seen, for example, as abdominal distension or as more generalised swelling in the form of widespread pitting oedema.

OVERALL IMPRESSION OF THE PATIENT
Start by deciding if there definite signs or symptoms of circulatory failure (i.e. abnormal vital signs, and/or any indicators of organ failure – e.g. brain or kidney dysfunction).

> **Key Point**
>
> If the patient is seriously unwell – i.e. there is evidence of impending or actual organ failure, or there is a high risk of deterioration – seek immediate assistance from someone with competence in the management of acute illness or critical care. If you are unsure, get help anyway.

Review the information you have gained and consider:

- *Can you be reasonably certain that the patient's blood volume adequate, or is it likely that he is hypovolaemic?*
  Remember that hypovolaemia is *very* common, especially in new admissions, but also amongst inpatients. Fluid overload is possible, but less common.
- *Is it probable that the heart is able to pump sufficient blood flow – assuming there is enough blood volume in the first instance – or is acute and/or chronic heart disease a potential issue?*
  - Does the patient have risk factors for heart disease: smoking, hypertension, raised cholesterol, obesity, inactivity, stress; diabetes; family history, etc? Increasing age is also a risk factor.
  - Are there signs and symptoms of cardiac ischaemia or acute myocardial infarction (see section titled 'Myocardial infarction' above)? A 12-lead ECG must be done as a matter of priority if heart disease is suspected; or if the pulse is irregular.
- *Is the systemic circulation abnormally constricted (and therefore increasing cardiac workload) or dilated (contributing to hypotension)?*
- *Is the heart rate so fast or so slow that cardiac output may be compromised?*

Another way of thinking about what is wrong and what needs to be done is to consider any of the common causes of circulatory collapse that might be relevant.

SHOCK
The term 'shock' is used to describe severe circulatory failure that results in body tissues having insufficient oxygen to function properly, and then to organ failure. This is usually due to inadequate oxygen delivery, although sometimes there is an additional problem to do with cells' inability to take up and use oxygen even when it is available.

There are several different types of shock (see Table 6.4). Shock states are generally marked by hypotension and compensatory tachycardia (and tachypnoea). However, differences between other aspects of the patient presentation can help

Table 6.4 Types of shock: summary

	Pulse	Peripheral circulation, central (neck) veins	Fluid therapy required	Other considerations
Hypovolaemic shock – haemorrhage, – severe dehydration	Weak, thready	Cool, constricted peripheries; increased diastolic BP	Definitely	Remember that there can be considerable internal fluid losses
Distributive shock Septic shock; Anaphylactic shock; Neurogenic shock	May be normal or large volume, 'bounding'	Warm, dilated peripheries; decreased diastolic BP	Definitely	Vasodilation may be so great that fluid resuscitation alone cannot increase venous return enough to generate an adequate BP a vasoconstrictor such as noradrenaline may be required
Cardiogenic shock – acute MI, – acute heart failure	Weak, thready	Cool, constricted peripheries; increased diastolic BP Neck veins likely to be distended (raised jugular venous pressure)	Possibly	The heart can simply be too weak to pump blood through an excessively constricted circulation; vasodilator therapy may be indicated, with perhaps a diuretic to reduce the fluid load on the heart
Obstructive shock – pulmonary embolism, – tension pneumothorax, – cardiac tamponade	Weak, thready	Cool, constricted peripheries, increased diastolic BP Neck veins likely to be distended (raised jugular venous pressure)	Probably	There may not be a problem with the heart itself as such; therefore, fluid is probably needed to optimise the pumping of blood past and around the obstruction

distinguish between the various causes of severe circulatory failure and therefore guide treatment.

- *Hypovolaemic shock* (lack of blood volume) can be caused by haemorrhage (internal or external) or severe dehydration, with typical signs and symptoms as described above (i.e. hypotension, tachycardia, a weak thready pulse, cool peripheries, and a raised diastolic BP).
- *Cardiogenic shock* (sometimes termed 'pump failure') is most often caused by myocardial infarction or other problems with the heart itself (e.g. acute decompensation of chronic heart failure, severe valvular disease, gross cardiac arrhythmias). Signs and symptoms may be similar to those of hypovolaemia (i.e. weak pulse, cool peripheries), except that because the heart is less able to pump blood into the systemic circulation, any blood returning to the heart tends to accumulate in the veins leading into the heart and the pulmonary circulation. This congestion may be revealed by distended neck veins and signs and symptoms of excess fluid in the lungs (pulmonary oedema): dyspnoea, reduced oxygen saturation, and crackles heard in the lungs.
- *Septic shock* is caused by infection and a systemic inflammatory response. Again, hypotension and tachycardia are usually present. However, in this instance, a normal or large volume pulse may be felt, and the peripheries may be warm and pink – with a low diastolic BP – as the inflammatory response tends to vasodilate. *Anaphylactic shock* (a severe systemic allergic reaction – e.g. to certain drugs, foods, insect stings) presents with a similar cardiovascular picture. *Neurogenic shock* also involves vasodilation, caused by damage to the central nervous system that reduces autonomic enervation of the systemic circulation. Without sympathetic nervous impulses to regulate arterial tone, vasodilation occurs and blood pressure falls. Septic, anaphylactic and neurogenic shock are sometimes grouped together under the heading '*distributive shock*'. This description makes the point that in these conditions the heart itself may be more or less undamaged and even that the volume of blood in the circulation may not necessarily be greatly reduced. Rather, changes in vascular tone alter the

normal distribution of blood flow to vital organs and the overall (blood) pressure in the system tends to fall.

- *Obstructive shock* is caused by some mechanism that prevents or greatly reduces the flow of blood through the heart and pulmonary vessels, such as massive pulmonary embolism (PE), tension pneumothorax, cardiac tamponade, or severe aortic stenosis. Once more, hypotension and tachycardia are usually found, with cool peripheries and raised diastolic BP associated with vasoconstriction. Some of these patients will also have pulmonary congestion and distended neck veins, depending on the exact location and severity of the obstruction. PE and tension pneumothorax are sometimes labelled as forms of cardiogenic shock, but the problems in these cases are not to do with the heart itself and different approaches to treatment are required.

Note that the distinctions between different types of shock are not completely clear-cut. For example, severe dehydration and hypovolaemic shock can be caused by diarrhoea, vomiting and other sorts of gastrointestinal loss. Diarrhoea and vomiting is often due to infection, so there may be a degree of sepsis too. Furthermore, gastrointestinal loss can lead to gross electrolyte imbalance causing arrhythmias and even cardiogenic shock in extreme cases. Likewise, severe sepsis may not actually reduce the volume of blood in the cardiovascular system as such, but gross vasodilation causes what is termed a relative hypovolaemia. However, sepsis also usually causes capillary leak as the blood vessels become more permeable, so fluid *is* lost from the circulation. Nonetheless, examination of the pulse, the tone of the peripheral circulation, and the condition of the veins – particularly central veins – can usually help clarification of the main problem. Each cause of circulatory failure has its own particular treatment options (e.g. surgery for haemorrhage from a specific bleeding point, antibiotics for sepsis, thrombolysis for myocardial infarction and pulmonary embolism). The shocked patient always needs an expert review to make such decisions, but just as important in the first instance is deciding how best to optimise blood flow and blood pressure. This usually involves fluid therapy.

Another approach is to structure a patient evaluation using what resuscitation experts call the '4 Hs and 4 Ts': common, potentially reversible causes of collapse. That is, the patient history and examination may point to one or other of:

- **H**ypoxia
- **H**ypovolaemia (e.g. haemorrhage – or severe dehydration, diarrhoea/vomiting, severe sepsis)
- **H**ypo/**H**yperkalaemia (low/high serum potassium) – or hypoglycaemia, hypocalcaemia (low serum calcium), low pH; or other metabolic disorder,
- **H**ypothermia
- **T**ension pneumothorax
- Cardiac **T**amponade
- **T**oxins (i.e. poisoning – including medications: review the drug chart)
- **T**hrombosis – or embolism – in the pulmonary, coronary, or cerebral circulation.

(Resuscitation Council UK, 2006).

BLOOD SAMPLING

Patients with actual or potential acute illness require certain blood tests (especially if they have newly deteriorated), many of which reflect or influence various aspects of cardiovascular function. That is:

- Urea and electrolytes, creatinine
- Full blood count
- Clotting studies
- Liver function tests and amylase may be indicated too, particularly if an acute abdominal problem has been identified.

A sample for 'group and save' (blood group identified and serum checked for antibodies) should be taken if it is thought that blood transfusion might be required; or for cross-matching if transfusion is likely.

Some important blood tests for the patient in circulatory failure may need to be requested separately from the usual ones (e.g. serum calcium and magnesium, and C-reactive protein). Potassium, calcium and magnesium are all particularly important in cardiac function: abnormal levels cause arrhythmias and even cardiac arrest. Sodium, potassium, calcium and magnesium levels in patients in acute circulatory failure should always be checked, with a request to get the results urgently. Bicarbonate (in the form of total carbon dioxide (Total CO_2)) and especially serum lactate are useful markers of the adequacy of tissue perfusion, but usually need to be specifically requested: in septic patients, an initial lactate of ≥ 4.0 mmol/l is correlated with a high risk of death. Bicarbonate and sometimes lactate may also be measured from an arterial blood sample if taken in hospitals with the appropriate equipment.

If the patient is believed to have severe sepsis, two sets of blood cultures are required to aid identification of the causative microorganism: that is, two pairs of blood culture bottles (Dellinger et al, 2008).

Key Point

If a number of blood samples are to be collected, blood cultures should be taken first in order to reduce the risk of contamination. Sputum, urine and any other potentially infected body fluid or tissue should be sent to microbiology as well.

Not all ward staff are trained in phlebotomy. However, blood tests provide crucial data in acute illness. If the practitioner is unable to obtain the samples her/himself, s/he should at least get the bottles and blood collection equipment ready for when help arrives so as to minimise delay.

NEXT STEPS

Venous access is vital for optimal management of acute illness. It may be that the patient already has several intravenous cannulae: these should have been identified during the physical examination. Any cannulae must be known to be patent and free of complications such as phlebitis. If this is not the case, at least one but preferably two short, large-diameter cannulae (ideally 14G (brown or orange) or16G (grey)) should be placed: if fluid resuscitation is needed, these cannulae can accommodate more than twice the flow-rate of more narrow cannulae (18G or smaller). Blood sampling from newly inserted cannulae can be done too. As before, if the initial assessor is not trained in cannulation, the necessary equipment can be got ready for when help arrives.

DECIDING ON FIRST-LINE TREATMENT

Any problems with airway, breathing, ventilation and oxygenation should already have been dealt with by this stage. Then, if any reversible causes of circulatory collapse have been identified, there may be specific treatments required, such as surgery to control bleeding, electrolyte replacement or removal, needle decompression and chest drain placement for tension pneumothorax, antidotes or other supportive therapy for poisoning. Expert help will probably be needed for these interventions.

Crucially, intravenous fluid therapy – or fluid resuscitation – is a priority in almost all forms of severe circulatory failure (see Table 6.4 above: 'Types of shock: summary'). Nonetheless, clinicians are sometimes anxious about giving large volumes of fluid, even to obviously hypotensive patients, usually for fear of 'overloading' the cardiovascular system.

The fluid challenge

One way of clarifying the situation is to use a closely observed 'fluid challenge' as an assessment tool as well as a treatment. Any possible risks can be minimised by careful monitoring before, during and after the process. If key vital signs improve with fluids, then it is unlikely that the patient is overloaded; indeed, further fluid is probably indicated. However, if any vital signs become more abnormal, it may be that the cardiovascular system is already adequately filled. Even if it turns out that this is the case, being sure that the patient is not hypovolaemic is an important piece of information: attention can then be focused on other causes of circulatory failure.

Fluid challenge is the technique of giving a large bolus of intravenous fluid (crystalloid or colloid) over a relatively short period – and, importantly, assessing the physiological response. For example, guidelines for management of patients with severe sepsis and suspected hypovolaemia suggest that 1000 ml of crystalloid or 300–500 ml colloid are given over 30 minutes as a starting point (Dellinger et al, 2008) – through two lines if necessary. Similar volumes are likely to be required in other forms of distributive shock, and in hypovolaemic shock.

Patients in obstructive shock and cardiogenic shock can be fluid depleted too – which requires treatment – but are also more at risk of fluid overload. Therefore, for these patients, it may be sensible to check the effects of a fluid challenge after, say, each 250 ml.

Steps in the fluid challenge

1. First, note baseline signs and symptoms, i.e.
   - Repiratory rate
   - Oxygen saturation,
   - Breath sounds – if possible. Note: there may be evidence of pulmonary oedema (e.g. crackles on ausculation) but the patient could still be hypovolaemic and in need of fluid replacement
   - Pulse rate, rhythm, volume
   - Peripheral perfusion (capillary refill, limb temperature)
   - Blood pressure
   - Consciousness,
   - Urine output – if possible; and central venous pressure – also if possible (see below).
2. Give the fluid – ≥ 250 ml if the circulatory failure might have a cardiogenic component, 500–1000 ml if it is obviously a case of hypovolaemic or distributive shock – in ≤30 minutes.
3. Recheck the baseline signs and symptoms – the expectation is that one or more will have improved.
   - Assess whether or not blood flow (e.g. peripheral perfusion), blood pressure and organ function have returned to normal or near-normal.
   - If normality has not been restored, and there are no adverse signs (e.g. a more abnormal pulse or respiratory rate, lower oxygen saturations or blood pressure), the fluid challenge should be repeated.
   - If there are adverse signs – i.e. worsening signs and symptoms – it may be that not enough fluid has been given (e.g.

bleeding is occurring faster than the rate of fluid challenge); or that the heart is overloaded (quite possible if oxygen saturations are worse or crackles in the lungs more wide-spread). The first possibility indicates that more fluid is needed, the second that fluid infusion should be stopped and the patient reassessed. Seek expert help.

JUGULAR VENOUS AND CENTRAL VENOUS PRESSURE

It has already been highlighted that cardiogenic and obstructive shock states are associated with raised pressures in the pulmo-nary circulation, which can be transmitted to the jugular veins in the neck, causing noticeable distension of those veins. The degree of distension can sometimes be measured: this is the jugular venous pressure, calculated as the vertical height from the sternal angle (head of sternomastoid) to the highest level of pulsation visible in the internal or external jugular veins when the patient lies at a 45° angle (Figure 6.3). Such pulsations are not normally seen at all (i.e. it is abnormal to have raised jugular venous pressure).

Better still, if the patient has a central venous catheter (CVC) inserted, the central venous pressure (CVP) can be measured. The CVP reflects the pressure in the veins as they enter the right atrium. It is often used as an indicator of blood volume although this can be misleading; the relationship between right heart pres-sures and intravascular volume is unpredictable and affected by many factors including the tone of the systemic circulation. However, CVP levels and especially changes in CVP – as the patient becomes unwell and/or treatments are given – are still a useful marker of whether or not there is likely to be enough venous return to generate an adequate cardiac output. Measurement with a fluid manometer – as usually used in general wards – gives a typical value of 0–12 cm H_2O. Areas with more sophisticated equipment may use an electronic transducer which measures pressure in mm Hg, giving a normal range of about 0–9 mmHg (1 mmHg = 1.36 cm H_2O). Monitoring of CVP over time and especially in response to therapies such as a fluid chal-lenge is more important than the absolute value. It can help identify heart failure, and also obstructions to right ventricular outflow such as pulmonary embolus or cardiac tamponade.

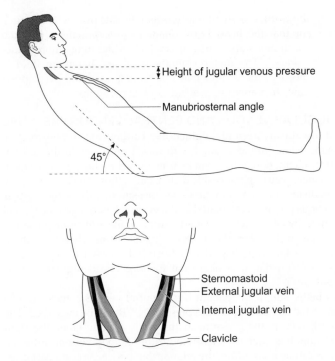

Fig. 6.3 The jugular veins
From Cox C, Physical Assessment for Nurses, copyright 2004 with permission of Blackwell Publishing

CVP is raised by:

- Left and/or right heart failure
- Right heart valve disease
- Fluid overload
- Pulmonary vascular hypertension or embolism
- Cardiac tamponade, pericarditis
- Increased intrathoracic pressure (e.g. due to haemothorax, pneumothorax, severe asthma, chronic obstructive pulmonary disease)

- Abdominal 'splinting' (e.g. pregnancy, ascites)
- Increased venous tone (e.g. sympathetic nervous stimulation).

    CVP is lowered by:

- Hypovolaemia
- Systemic vasodilation (e.g. septic shock, vasodilator overdose, sympathetic nervous dysfunction)
- Regional analgesia (e.g. epidural analgesia).

CVP measurement with a water manometer

The system consists of a bag of intravenous fluid – usually sodium chloride 0.9% ('normal saline') – and a fluid administration set connected to the CVC, with an upright manometer attached to the administration set by a three-way tap. The manometer's upper end is protected by a filter that ensures the sterility of the system. The manometer should be mounted on a measured scale. (See Figure 6.4.)

Measurement must be taken from a constant baseline, level with the right atrium. The patient should be consistently positioned as venous return may be reduced in an upright position and increased when lying flat. It is sometimes said that an accurate CVP can only be obtained with the patient is flat. However, as long as the measurement is always done with the patient in the *same* position, it is acceptable (and often preferable) to have the patient sitting up. Lateral (side-lying) positions obscure the relationship between the right atrium, the CVC tip, and the measurement baseline. Note that CVP may be artificially raised through infusion of fluids through the CVC while measurements are recorded, so any infusions should be briefly stopped during the process.

CVP measurement procedure

1. First, ensure that the normal saline is able to flow freely through the administration set and the CVC.
2. Position the patient comfortably: supine for greatest accuracy, but semi-recumbent/upright if too unstable to lie flat.
3. Determine the point on the manometer that is level with the right atrium (i.e. level with a point in the midaxillary line at

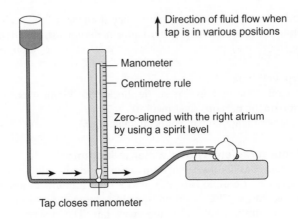

Direction of fluid flow when tap is in various positions

Manometer

Centimetre rule

Zero-aligned with the right atrium by using a spirit level

Tap closes manometer

The fluid level finally settles and oscillates with the respirations. The CVP is then the number of centimetres above or below zero

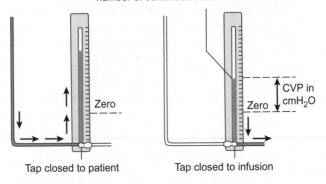

Zero

Tap closed to patient

Zero

CVP in cmH₂O

Tap closed to infusion

Fig. 6.4 CVP measurement with a water manometer
From Dougherty L, Lister S, The Royal Marsden Hospital Manual of Clinical Procedures (7th edn). Copyright 2008, reproduced with permission of Blackwell Publishing Ltd and The Royal Marsden Hospital

the fourth intercostal space). It is useful to mark the specific point on the midaxillary line, if the patient is agreeable. A spirit level may be used to establish the baseline point on the manometer scale. The scale itself can be adjusted so that the 'zero' point is aligned level with the right atrium.

4. Turn the three-way tap at the base of the manometer off to the patient, so that fluid from the administration set fills the manometer to a level well above the anticipated CVP (e.g. several centimetres more than 12 cm above the baseline). (However, the filter at the upper end of the manometer should not be made wet.)

5. Turn the three-way tap off to the administration set, and observe the fluid in the manometer (which should fall quite rapidly). Ensure that the fluid does not drop right to the bottom of the manometer as this could cause an air embolism to enter the system. If this seems possible, close the three-way tap to the manometer, and reposition the manometer lower on its stand before restarting the procedure.

6. The CVP can be read when the fluid falls no further (although it may fluctuate or 'swing' with respiration; in which case, take the measurement at the top of the swing). Again, consistency is important.

7. Turn the three-way tap off to the manometer, so that the fluid infusion gives a slow continuous flush through the CVC.

8. Reposition the patient comfortably as required.

9. Document the measurement on 'vital signs chart'.

Careful interpretation of the CVP is required – and should always be considered in conjunction with other parameters. A low CVP does not necessarily mean that the patient is hypovolaemic, and a high CVP may not mean that they are overloaded.

The fluid challenge and the CVP

If the vascular compartment is well filled with blood, the addition of a fluid bolus would usually be expected to noticeably increase the CVP, irrespective – for example – of whether the baseline measurement is 5, 10, 15 or 20 cm H_2O. As a general rule, if the CVP increases by 3 cm H_2O or more (> 2 mmHg) after a fluid challenge, it is likely that there is an adequate venous return to the heart. If the CVP does not increase by 3 cm H_2O (2 mm Hg), further fluid is probably required to optimise cardiac output.

CARDIAC MONITORING (ECG MONITORING)

It is beyond the scope of this book to detail the recording and interpretation of a 12-lead ECG, although this is an essential procedure in any acute illness where there may be cardiac involvement. A 12-lead ECG is particularly important in the proper diagnosis of rhythm abnormalities and acute coronary syndrome/myocardial infarction.

However, it is not uncommon for ward patients to have continuous cardiac monitoring. For example:

- if the patient has reported chest pain (angina)
- during recovery from an episode of acute heart failure or acute coronary syndrome
- if abnormal heart rates (bradycardia or tachycardia) or an irregular pulse have already been identified (these might be associated with fainting or collapse)
- if treatments are being given that can induce changes in heart rate or rhythm (e.g. infusion of electrolytes, insertion of a central venous catheter).

Setting up the cardiac monitor

The simplest of these machines have three leads (wires). Three adhesive electrodes each connected to one of the three leads from the monitor should be placed on the patient's chest: one below the right shoulder (RA, red lead), one below the left shoulder (LA, yellow lead), and one on the left lower chest/left upper area of the abdomen (LL, green lead). Ideally, electrodes should be placed over bone (see Figure 6.5). It may be necessary to shave chest hair in order to place the electrodes.

Up to 12 different views of the heart are possible if a 12-lead ECG is recorded, but for continuous monitoring the system is usually set up to view one of the positive leads (generally Lead II), meaning that most of the pattern of waveforms is seen above the isoelectric baseline (Figure 6.6).

The horizontal axis on the monitor equates to time, although it can be difficult to be certain about time spans unless a rhythm

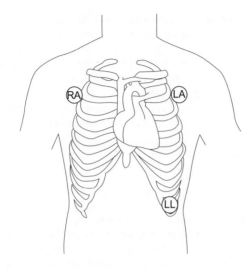

Fig. 6.5 Basic three-lead cardiac monitoring

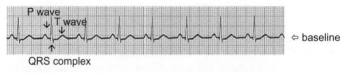

There is a pattern of regular, evenly spaced tall complexes.
Most of the pattern is seen above the isoelectric baseline.

Fig. 6.6 Normal 'sinus' rhythm: heart rate about 80/minute
From Jevon P, ECGs for Nurses, copyright 2003 with permission of Blackwell Publishing Ltd

strip is printed out. Each of the larger squares on the rhythm strip represents 0.2 (one-fifth) of a second. There are 29 complete large squares in the example above and most of another one (i.e. roughly 30 squares in total), meaning that this strip is a recording of 6 seconds of time. There are eight tall QRS complexes to be seen (in 6 seconds), so the heart rate over a minute here is 80.

The vertical axis on the ECG shows the amount of electrical current (voltage) generated during different times in the cardiac cycle. In Figure 6.6, the QRS complex forms the tallest section, because it reflects current through the large mass ventricles. The QRS is preceded by the P wave, which is created by current through the smaller mass atria.

A rhythm strip from a cardiac monitor is not a substitute for a 12-lead ECG. However it is a useful assessment tool.

Reviewing a rhythm strip – ask:

- *Is there any electrical activity to be seen?*
  Clearly there should be (assuming that the patient is alive!); otherwise, check the monitor and leads.
- *How many QRS complexes are there in a minute?*
  This is the ventricular rate, which should be associated with an equal number of palpable pulses. Heart rates > 100/minute or < 60/minute are considered abnormal and require further investigation, while rates > 150/minute or < 40/minute may well be life-threatening.
- *Are the QRS complexes evenly spaced?*
  Irregular rhythms are likely to impair coordinated cardiac contraction and cardiac output, and may also become more irregular – and life-threatening.
- *Is the QRS complex a normal width or is it broader?*
  The QRS is normally less than half a large square across at its widest point (see Figure 6.6). Broader QRS complexes indicate that conduction through the heart is not following the normal pathway. Again, such rhythms have the potential to reduce cardiac output. (See Figure 6.7.)

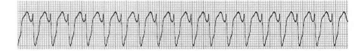

Fig. 6.7 Abnormally wide QRS complexes: heart rate about 180/minute (ventricular tachycardia: life threatening!)
From Jevon P, ECGs for Nurses, copyright 2003 with permission of Blackwell Publishing Ltd

- *Can a normal looking P wave be identified prior to each QRS complex?*

  As seen in Figure 6.6, P waves arise from normal conduction from the sino-atrial node (the heart's intrinsic pacemaker) through the atria. Altered or absent P waves may mean that the atria do not contract as they should (see Figure 6.8 below – atrial fibrillation, the most common dysrhythmia).

- *If there is an identifiable P wave? How is it related to the QRS complex?*

  Normally, each P wave is followed at a brief and unchanging interval by a QRS complex, illustrating conduction from the atria through to the ventricles. The period from the beginning of the P wave to the beginning of the QRS complex is usually no longer than 0.2 second (or one large square). This is called the PR interval. A longer PR interval indicates that 'heart

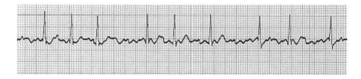

Fig. 6.8 Irregularly spaced but normal width QRS complexes; no P waves
From Jevon P, ECGs for Nurses, copyright 2003 with permission of Blackwell Publishing Ltd

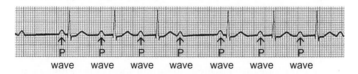

Fig. 6.9 P waves, followed at increasing intervals by normal width QRS complexes, until one QRS is missed entirely. The 4th P wave does not trigger a QRS – the impulse is blocked. Another P wave has to be generated first. (This is known as second-degree atrioventricular block – Mobitz Type I.)
From Jevon P, ECGs for Nurses, copyright 2003 with permission of Blackwell Publishing Ltd

block' may be occurring (i.e. disruption or even complete stoppage of conduction from the atria to the ventricles): see Figure 6.9 for examples of gradually increasing PR intervals.

Key Point

The most important question — irrespective of the ECG pattern – is of course: how is the patient?!

Further information can be gained by looking at the ST segment and T wave that usually follows the QRS – see Figure 6.6 'Normal sinus rhythm'. A different appearance such as a depressed or an elevated ST segment need not be sinister, but is worth discussing with someone experienced in viewing ECGs: these changes may be signs of myocardial ischaemia or infarction.

SUMMARY

A functioning heart and circulatory system is essential to deliver oxygen and nutrients to the tissues and remove waste products. However, chronic cardiovascular diseases and acute circulatory failure are frequent and often serious problems. Patient assessment should always include, as a minimum, looking at, talking to and listening to the patient; feeling the pulse, checking peripheral perfusion (peripheral temperature, capillary refill); and measuring blood pressure – as well as urine output if possible. These signs and symptoms should then be evaluated so as to decide whether or not the patient's blood volume and blood flow are likely to be adequate; whether or not there is sufficient haemoglobin in the system (and the haemoglobin is sufficiently saturated with oxygen); and whether or not the blood pressure is adequate. It is important to identify whether or not any body organ symptoms are affected: the brain, heart and kidneys are particularly sensitive to reductions in blood flow. Common causes of circulatory failure include hypovolaemia (which may be due to sepsis) and acute coronary syndrome/myocardial infarction. Fluid resuscitation is a priority in almost all forms of severe circulatory failure: early treatment is crucial.

CHAPTER 6: SCENARIOS

Scenario 6.1

A 24-year-old woman with a 3-day history of abdominal pain, diarrhoea and vomiting has just been admitted to the acute admissions ward from the Accident and Emergency department.

The patient arrives with 2 l/minute oxygen being given through a 'standard' face mask. She looks pink and slightly sweaty. She can be heard talking in sentences but is incoherent. She is visibly breathing fast.

Q 1 What would you assess?

The patient is talking in complete sentences – and has already been identified to be breathing – so the airway must be patent.

The respiratory rate is 34 breaths/minute. Both sides of the chest are moving, and auscultation reveals that there is good air entry throughout the lung fields with no abnormal sounds. The oxygen saturation is 100% on 2 l/minute oxygen (equivalent to about 28% oxygen).

Q 2 If the chest seems to be clear and the oxygen saturation is not low, why might she be breathing fast?

The patient's hands feel warm and a little sweaty. The capillary refill time is normal. The pulse rate is 120 beats/minute, feels regular and is thready (low volume). The blood pressure is 85/45 mm Hg. It is unclear whether or not the patient has passed urine since arriving at the hospital. There is no urinary catheter.

Q 3 Have any issues arisen that require immediate treatment?

Q 4 The diastolic blood pressure is also low – what does this indicate?

Q 5 What needs to be done?

Q 6 What else should be done at this point?

Q 7 Which blood tests should be requested?

The main problem – to be treated as a matter of priority – is acute circulatory failure: indeed, this patient may be in shock (due to hypovolaemia and sepsis). Aggressive intravenous fluid resuscitation should be commenced and the rapid assessment process completed by review of Disability and Everything else.

The patient is opening her eyes from time to time; she is not alert but responds to voice and therefore recorded as V on the AVPU scale (see Chapter 7). This is a reduced level of consciousness – and a cause for concern – but should not affect the patient's ability to maintain a patent airway.

Q 8 Why might there be a reduced level of consciousness?

Further inspection of the patient does not reveal any other obvious abnormalities, except that the abdomen is tender to touch (the patient grimaces). The patient's temperature is 37.7°C.

Q 9 An arterial blood gas is taken: the results are as below – what do these values signify?

pH	7.15	(normal range 7.35–7.45)
pCO_2	2.9 kPa	(normal range 4.6–6.1 kPa)
HCO_3^-	7.5 mmol/l	(normal range 22–26 mmol/l)
pO_2	18.5 kPa on 28% oxygen	

Q 10 What are the causes of this metabolic acidosis?

Answers to scenario 6.1

Q1 As always, Airway–Breathing–Circulation–Disability–Everything else (A–B–C–D–E).

Q2 There may be several reasons, including brain injury (which may be identified when Disability is assessed, although the fact that she is talking makes massive brain injury unlikely), anxiety or pain. Alternatively – and very commonly – she may be hyperventilating in order to compensate for a metabolic acidosis by eliminating more carbon dioxide than normal. This could be tested in due course with blood gas analysis (preferably using arterial blood): metabolic acidosis is indicated by a low bicarbonate value.

Q3 It has been established that the airway is patent, the chest is clear and the patient is well oxygenated: breathing is abnormal, but this does not seem to be a case of respiratory failure (oxygenation is satisfactory and CO_2 is not likely to be high with fast breathing and a clear chest, although the CO_2 should be checked in due course). Therefore, the patient's breathing does not require further support at this stage, other than being facilitated by helping the patient sit up. However, there are signs of significant circulatory failure. The systolic BP is low: some healthy young people may have a systolic pressure at this level, but the patient is also tachycardic so this is not a normal state. Expert advice is required as a matter of urgency. A 12-lead ECG should also be requested (to check the nature of the tachycardia already identified) – but completion of the assessment process should not be delayed by this: therefore, more help is needed.

Q4 Low diastolic pressure – and the warm peripheries already felt – are indicative of a process of vasodilatation (e.g. due to inflammation, infection (sepsis) or anaphylaxis).

Q5 Fluid resuscitation is required in most cases of circulatory failure (see Types of shock: summary table, page 124). Cardiogenic shock is the main exception to this general rule, but is usually associated with cool peripheries and an increased diastolic BP – which are not evident in this instance. Consequently, the priority is to establish venous access (if not already done) and to give one or more fluid challenges in order to restore the circulating volume and normalise the blood pressure.

Q6 Unless blood tests have been done within the last 2 hours, cannulation is also an opportunity to take bloods for laboratory analysis. If it is unclear if, when, or which bloods have already been taken, a new set of samples should be anyway obtained.

Q7 Urea and electrolytes, creatinine, full blood count, clotting studies, liver function tests, amylase (remembering that the patient presented with an acute abdominal problem), blood glucose, calcium, magnesium, C-reactive protein and two sets of blood cultures – the patient has signs of sepsis (as well as a history of diarrhoea and vomiting, which may well be due to gastrointestinal infection). Serum lactate measurement, from a venous blood sample (or an arterial blood sample if possible), should be obtained too.

Q8 Consciousness is discussed in detail in Chapter 7; but at this point the most likely explanation is that there is reduced cerebral blood flow and therefore reduced cerebral oxygenation due to hypotension. For completeness, the pupillary reflexes should be checked and a bedside blood glucose measurement obtained.

Q9 This is a severe metabolic acidosis (both the pH and the bicarbonate are very low). The patient is hyperventilating in an effort to compensate (as indicated by the very low pCO_2), but is still acidaemic. She is oxygenating well (the pO_2 is high); indeed, the pO_2 would probably still be in the normal range even without oxygen therapy. (N.b. she is getting 2 l/minute oxygen through a 'standard' face mask: these are designed to have $\geq$5 l/minute flow; nasal cannulae should be used instead.)

Q10 Possible causes include loss of bicarbonate in profuse diarrhoea, acute renal failure (to be confirmed by measurement of urine output and serum creatinine) and tissue hypoxia due to inadequate circulation (diagnosis may be supported by a raised lactate level).

Summary

This patient has acute circulatory failure due to hypovolaemia caused by prolonged diarrhoea and vomiting and – almost certainly – sepsis. Inadequate circulation is indicated by hypotension, tachycardia and deterioration in brain function. The patient is at risk of acute renal failure too (urine output and blood results need to be checked). Fluid resuscitation is the priority, aiming, in the first instance, to bring the systolic blood pressure up to at least 90 mm Hg, and the heart rate down: it is very possible that at least 1–2 l of fluid will be required in the first 1–2 hours. The patient should be catheterised in order to monitor urine output, with the objective that at least 0.5 ml/kg of body weight per hour is produced. The second priority in this case is administration of intravenous broad spectrum antibiotics (if this has not already been done): the standard is that antibiotics should be given within 3 hours for Accident and Emergency admissions and 1 hour for ward patients. Finally, consider whether there are adequate resources available in the area to manage this patient: she will require re-assessment of Airway, Breathing, Circulation, Disability and Everything else; frequent measurement of vital signs and urine output; maintenance of oxygen therapy and intravenous fluids; and all nursing care.

Scenario 6.2

You are caring for a 62-year-old man on the first day following an emergency Hartmann's procedure, i.e. surgical resection of a large colorectal tumour that had been causing acute bowel obstruction. He is overweight and has a history of hypertension and angina. The patient has been complaining of pain for much of the time since the operation, despite his repeated use of a patient-controlled analgesia system. He now looks agitated. When you come to record his vital signs, the patient is slumped in the bed. He is talking but seems confused.

You find that his temperature is 37.9°C, respiratory rate is 25 breaths/minute, oxygen saturation is 91% with the patient breathing air (his nasal cannulae have slipped off), pulse is 108 beats/minute and blood pressure is 105/53 mm Hg.

Q 1 What is your impression of the vital signs?

In this case, vital signs were last recorded 4 hours previously: the temperature then was 37.5 °C, respiratory rate 22 breaths/minute, oxygen saturation 96%, pulse 98 beats/minute and blood pressure 132/65 mm Hg.

Q 2 What would you do now?

As noted above, the patient is talking – although he is distracted and confused – so the airway must be patent. The respiratory rate is now 26 breaths/minute. You can see both sides of the chest moving, and, if auscultated, you can easily hear air entry in the upper lung zones (on both sides). However, sounds of air entry are quiet in the mid-zones and can barely be heard at all in the lower zones. There are a few scattered crackle sounds. You also notice that the patient's abdomen seems very distended. It is quite difficult to get a consistent signal displayed on the pulse oximeter, but you eventually record an oxygen saturation of 93% on 4 l/minute oxygen (equivalent to about 36% oxygen).

Q 3 The patient obviously has some breathing problems – the respiratory rate is increasing, oxygen saturations have deteriorated from earlier in the day and there is reduced – or absent air entry – in the lower part of the chest. Crackle sounds may be signs of secretions or fluid in small airways. What would you do next?

The patient does cough when asked – albeit quite weakly. The oxygen saturation subsequently increases to 94%, but the nature of the crackles does not change.

You already know the heart rate and blood pressure (which has dropped), and that it is difficult to get a good signal on the oximeter.

- The patient's hands are cool and clammy.
- You palpate a radial pulse and find that it is fast, feels regular but is 'thready'.
- Capillary refill time is 5 seconds.
- Urine output was last recorded on the fluid chart 4 hours previously: it was written that the catheter bag

was emptied at that time, and there is 130 mL of urine now.

Q 4 What do these findings indicate?

Q 5 What should be done next?

Q 6 The arterial blood gas results are as follows – what do these values signify?

- pH   7.30   (normal range 7.35–7.45),

- pCO_2 4.2 kPa   (normal range 4.6–6.1 kPa),

- HCO_3^- 15.3 mmol/l   (normal range 22–26 mmol/l),

- pO_2 31.7 kPa, now on 50% oxygen.

- The Hb is 9.3 g/dl. In addition the serum lactate is measured at 4.2 mmol/l.

Q 7 So, should the patient be given a fluid challenge – or not?

Answers to scenario 6.2

Q1 None of the vital signs are grossly deranged, and on some track and trigger systems would not reach a level to trigger a call to a doctor or Outreach. However, five signs are at least a little abnormal, with the confusion, respiratory rate and oxygen saturation perhaps the most concerning. Even the BP is worth thinking about: a systolic BP of 105 mm Hg would not be unusual in a fit young person, but 62-year-old men average a systolic BP of 137 mm Hg; furthermore, this particular 62-year-old man has a history of high blood pressure. In addition, a heart rate above systolic BP is in itself abnormal. Vital signs should always be considered in context, i.e. if possible, you should check if these values are better, worse – or the same – as previous recordings.

Q2 The temperature, respiratory rate, oxygen saturation and heart rate are all more abnormal than they were before, and the blood pressure has markedly decreased. You should get some help to sit the patient more upright, re-apply the nasal cannulae (or use a mask) to improve oxygen saturation – turning up the flow rate in order to get a rapid improvement and then proceed with a full A–B–C–D–E assessment.

Q3 An immediate referral for urgent assessment by a doctor (ideally, someone from the surgical team) and/or the Outreach team is in order – you should emphasise that the patient may have been unwell for several hours, has signs of worsening respiratory function, adverse cardio-vascular signs (tachycardia, falling blood pressure) and a deterioration in mental function. Review by a physiother-apist would be useful too. You should ask the patient to cough so as to see if a) he can understand and obey com-mands, b) it improves the oxygen saturation and c) if it helps eliminate the crackle sounds.

You should ask a colleague to ensure that help is coming. You have optimised the patient's position so as to enable him to breathe with least difficulty, and the oxygen saturation is at a safe level – at least for the time being. It is noteworthy that the crackles were not affected by coughing: secretions may be displaced by coughing but fluid in the lungs (pulmonary oedema) may not. A chest x-ray would be helpful in due course, but at this point there is probably nothing more you can do with regard to the patient's breathing, so you should continue the A–B–C–D–E assessment and proceed to assess the Circulation in more detail.

Q4 They confirm that the circulation is significantly compro-mised. The pulse is low volume and the peripheries are poorly perfused (you might check the temperature of the patient's feet at this point too). If the peripheries are under-perfused, it is likely that vital organs will also be compromised: the reduced level of consciousness may be one indicator of this. Furthermore, if the patient is of an average or above average body weight (i.e. >83 kg), you would expect at least 170 mL urine in 4 hours. As this patient is overweight, it is likely that his renal function has also been affected (which is most often due to under-perfusion in this sort of case). In other words, you have already established that the patient has problems in the lungs and circulatory system, and that cerebral function and renal function seem to be deteriorating too, i.e. four organ systems are showing signs of failure – the patient is seriously ill (and quite possibly critically ill). He needs immediate review by a senior doctor, and, ideally, a critical care specialist.

Q5 Treatment of acute circulatory failure is a priority, requiring good quality venous access, i.e. at least one and preferably two large diameter cannulae. Potential causes of circulatory failure should be considered (think about the types of shock or 4 Hs and 4 Ts described in the Circulation chapter). If the patient's history is known – as in this case – it is possible to focus on the most likely causes. He has angina (from coronary heart disease), and has had recent major surgery. Common complications of major surgery do include respiratory failure (e.g. from chest infection, or pulmonary embolism) and circulatory failure (e.g. due to bleeding or dysrhythmias or acute coronary syndrome/ myocardial function – leading to heart failure or thromboembolis), renal failure, infection and sepsis. Therefore, the patient may be developing hypovolaemic, cardiogenic, septic (distributive) or obstructive shock!

This is a difficult situation, but you can ask the following questions to clarify what is happening (remembering that this needs to be a rapid process):

i) Is the patient's blood volume adequate, or might he be hypovolaemic?

There are certainly clinical signs of hypovolaemia. You could also enquire about what happened during surgery with regard to blood loss and replacement, and overall fluid balance (a member of the surgical team should have arrived by this time), then check the ward fluid charts to see what has happened since. It should be remembered that there is likely to have been considerable unmeasured fluid losses. In this case, the patient is said to have left Theatre recovery in a more-or-less neutral balance and has subsequently received 100 ml/hour maintenance fluid (bearing in mind that he weighs approximately 100 kg). This sort of regimen would not usually result in fluid overload. A pulmonary embolism obstructing blood flow through the pulmonary circulation is also possible, but although the patient has a worsening oxygen saturation, it has not decreased so much as to suggest a massive embolism.

ii) Is it probable that the heart is able to pump properly?

He has a history of angina and has been complaining of pain (though not obviously chest pain); certainly acute on chronic heart failure is a possibility. It would be useful to try and assess the jugular veins – which may be distended in heart failure (and pulmonary embolism) but not in hypovolaemia. However, in this case – with an obese patient – it may not be possible to visualise the jugular veins at all.

A 12-lead ECG could reveal whether there were signs of acute ischaemia, which would be indicative of possible acute heart failure (as would the pulmonary crackles). In this case, it transpires that there are new changes on the ECG.

iii) Is the systemic circulation abnormally constricted or dilated?

It is certainly not dilated: the peripheries are cold. Therefore, the hypotension is not due to vasodilation.

iv) Is the heart rate so fast, so slow or so irregular that cardiac output may be compromised?

This is not likely with a regular rhythm and pulse of 108.

v)   Is the haemoglobin concentration sufficient?

Given the fact of major surgery, and then an acute deterioration, bleeding is a possibility. Continuation of the assessment – D and E(xposure) – should reveal any external bleeding, but internal haemorrhage is also quite possible in this case: the abdomen is very distended. The quickest way to get an Hb measure is often with a blood gas sample, which should therefore be taken. N.b. a normal Hb is not necessarily a sign that there is no bleeding, certainly in the first stages of haemorrhage.

Q6 This is a severe metabolic acidaemia: the pH and the HCO_3^- are low. The patient is hyperventilating to try and compensate as shown by the low pCO_2. The raised lactate fits with a diagnosis of poor perfusion – and possibly of ischaemic tissue (e.g. in the bowel). One positive is that the patient is well oxygenated, albeit on 50% oxygen. The Hb is below the normal range, and this is particularly important for a patient with heart disease. There may be some blood for transfusion left over after surgery, but if not, more blood should be ordered.

Q7 On balance, it is most likely that the patient is hypovolaemic, so monitored intravenous fluid resuscitation is needed, using Hartmann's or a colloid solution in the first instance. Five hundred millilitres could be given as a fluid challenge to start with, while further review of D and E is undertaken: the patient may well need to be taken back to surgery for re-laparotomy. If there is not a senior surgeon present as yet, referral should be escalated to an on-call senior as matter of great urgency.

RECOMMENDED READING

Powell-Tuck J, Gosling P, Lobo DN et al (2008) British Consensus Guidelines on Intravenous Fluid Therapy for Adult Surgical Patients. Intensive Care Society, London

REFERENCES

Bellomo R, Ronco C, Kellum JA, et al (2004) Acute renal failure – definition, outcome measures, animal models, fluid therapy and information technology needs: the Second International Consensus Conference of the Acute Dialysis Quality Initiative (ADQI) Group. Critical Care 8(4):R204–212

Dellinger RP, Levy MM, Carlet JM, et al (2008) Surviving Sepsis Campaign: International guidelines for management of severe sepsis and septic shock, 2008. Critical Care Medicine 36(1):296–327

Guyton AC, Hall JE (2006) Textbook of Medical Physiology (11th edn). Elsevier Saunders, Philadelphia

Hébert PC, Tinmouth A, Corwin HL (2007) Controversies in RBC transfusion in the critically ill. Chest 131(5):1583–1590

Information Centre (2006) Health Survey for England 2005: Latest Trends (Tables). NHS Information Centre (www.ic.nhs.uk/statistics-and-data-collections/healthand-lifestyles-related-surveys/health-survey-for-england/health-survey-for-england-2005-latest-trends)

Joly HR, Weil MH (1969) Temperature of the great toe as an indication of the severity of shock. Circulation 39(1):131–138

Levy MM, Fink MP, Marshall JC, et al (2003) 2001 SCCM/ESICM/ACCP/ATS/SIS International Sepsis Definitions Conference. Critical Care Medicine 31(4):1250–1256

Low D, Milne M (2007) Crystalloids, colloids, blood, blood products and blood substitutes. Anaesthia and Intensive Care Medicine 8(2):56–59

NICE (2006) Clinical Guideline CG34: Hypertension. National Institute for Health and Clinical Excellence, London

Pickering TG, Hall JE, Appel LJ et al 2005. Recommendations for blood pressure measurement in humans and experimental animals: Part 1: blood pressure measurement in humans: a statement for professionals from the Subcommittee of Professional and Public Education of the American Heart Association Council on High Blood Pressure Research. Hypertension 45(1):142–161

Resuscitation Council UK (2006) Advanced Life Support (5th edn). Resuscitation Council UK, London

Scarborough P, Allender S, Peto V, et al (2008) Regional and social differences in coronary heart disease 2008. British Heart Foundation, London

Thygesen K, Alpert JS, White HD, et al (2007) Universal definition of myocardial infarction. Circulation 116(22):2634–2653

UK Food Standards Agency: www.eatwell.gov.uk/healthydiet/nutritionessentials/vitaminsandminerals/sodiumchloride/

Vincent JL, Weil MH (2006) Fluid challenge revisited. Critical Care Medicine 34(5):1333–1337

A–B–C–**D**–E: Acute Neurological Care (Disability)

7

INTRODUCTION

This chapter discusses the assessment and initial treatment measures for acute neurological care, which corresponds with the disability (D) section of the A–B–C–D–E assessment model introduced in chapter 1. Disability is the description given to the neurological function of the patient. In previous chapters we have discussed the assessment of the patient using preceding steps of the A–B–C–D–E approach. Problems with the Airway, Breathing and Circulation have all been shown to have a potential adverse affect on conscious level, and it has been seen how initial treatment measures in A, B and C can prevent the patient's conscious level deteriorating. When assessing disability it is essential that A, B and C have been assessed first, and any immediate problems detected have been addressed.

The chapter will be divided into three main sections. The first is a brief overview of the neurological system, including basic anatomy and physiology, discussions about the implications of the impairment of the neurological system, major causes of reduction of conscious level and the different types of coma. The second section discusses neurological assessment techniques, concentrating on the Awake/Voice/Pain/Unresponsive (AVPU) system and Glasgow Coma Scale (GCS). Issues such as painful stimuli, pupil reaction and blood glucose levels will be discussed. The final section of this chapter examines some common investigations and the initial treatment of the neurologically compromised patient with specific conditions, as well as some nursing care advice. Case scenarios end the chapter, giving nurses a chance to test their own knowledge on assessing and treating the neurologically impaired patient.

The acutely ill general ward patient remains the focus of this chapter, with discussions of the types of situations and problems these patients and the nurses caring for them commonly face.

LEARNING OBJECTIVES

By the end of this chapter you should be able to:

❑ Recall the basic anatomy and physiology of the nervous system
❑ Describe the common causes of impaired conscious level
❑ Describe the types of coma
❑ Assess conscious level
❑ Describe the Glasgow Coma Scale
❑ Discuss some of the common neurological investigations
❑ Discuss the care of the patient with a reduced conscious level.

SECTION 1: ANATOMY AND PHYSIOLOGY, CAUSES AND TYPES OF COMA

Brief overview of neurological system

The neurological, or nervous system, controls everything we think, feel and do, and is the most complex and wide-reaching bodily system. A detailed description of the nervous system's anatomy and physiology is beyond the scope of this book, but a brief overview of the main functions of the nervous system will be presented here in order that the general ward nurse can relate basic anatomy and physiology to the fundamental aspects of an initial neurological assessment, apply knowledge to assessment findings, initiate appropriate treatment, and know when to get more expert help.

The components of the neurological system can be organised into three main systems, which consist of:

1. The *central nervous system* (brain; spinal cord)
2. The *peripheral nervous system* (peripheral nerves; cranial nerves)
3. The *autonomic nervous system* (sympathetic system; parasympathetic system).

The peripheral nervous system senses stimuli such as the touch of a cobweb on your arm, the smell of bacon, and a full bladder, as well as sensing changes in blood pH, blood glucose, or levels of oxygen. These stimuli are sent to the brain via the spinal cord, cranial nerves and autonomic system, where they are interpreted and translated into a response. Some responses are voluntary, such as wiping the cobweb from your arm, and some are involuntary, such as salivating to the smell of bacon. The involuntary responses to sensory stimuli are included in the autonomic nervous system, divided into the sympathetic and parasympathetic systems. The autonomic system regulates the activity of organs such as the heart, glands and smooth muscle.

The brain consists of four main parts: brain stem, cerebellum, diencephalon and cerebrum (Tortora and Grabowski, 2000). Different areas of the brain are responsible for receiving these messages via the peripheral nerves and autonomic system and organising the stimuli into a specific response. (Figure 7.1 shows the main areas.)

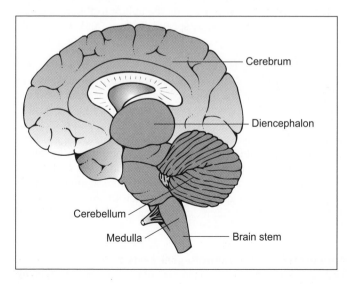

Fig. 7.1 The brain

- **The brain stem** connects the spinal cord to the diencephalon and consists of the medulla oblongata, pons and midbrain, vital for controlling breathing, heart rate and blood vessel tone, as well as the coordination of protective reactions such as coughing, gagging, vomiting and sneezing. Ten of the 12 cranial nerves emerge from the brain stem, which also contains the reticular activating system responsible for maintaining consciousness (Tortora and Grabowski, 2000).
- **The cerebellum** lies behind the brain stem, under the cerebrum and is responsible for smoothing and coordinating bodily movements, and regulating posture and balance.
- **The diencephalon** lies above the brain stem, between the brain stem and cerebrum. It contains the thalamus (which is responsible for relaying sensations such as pain, temperature and pressure, and plays a central role in awareness and cognition) and the hypothalamus (which is a major regulator of homeostasis, as well as organising hearing, taste and smell).
- **The cerebrum** is the largest part of the brain, sitting above the diencephalon, and gives us the ability to think, calculate, create, read, write and speak (Tortora and Grabowski, 2000).

On a basic level, the function of the neurological system is to ensure the continued survival of the organism, and make certain the propagation of the species. The nervous system works in harmony with the endocrine system to maintain homeostasis in the internal environment, as well as monitoring and responding to threats from the external environment. As neurological function deteriorates, then so does the body's ability to regulate its internal environment, and assess and respond to external threats. The range of risk to the patient can be from a minor sensory impairment, resulting in the development of pressure sores, to the loss of central systems controlling breathing, resulting in death.

Impairment of the neurological system
Impairment of the neurological system is common in the acutely ill patient. This impairment will generally be manifested in a

change in mental state, ranging from an altered personality or confusion to a reduction or loss of consciousness. Some of the causes of an impaired consciousness will have been discussed in previous chapters when discussing A, B and C. The main causes of impairment of consciousness can be grouped into seven broad categories outlined in Box 7.1.

Impairment of the nervous system may be permanent or temporary. Changes in mental state or conscious level are a major sign of deterioration in the general ward patient. In a study of 64 patients who suffered a cardiac arrest by Schein et al (1990), it was found that 54 (84%) patients had reported changes in behaviour in the 8 hours preceding the arrest. Other studies have found that a fall in conscious level is a significant factor in the signs preceding a cardiac arrest (Buist et al, 2004; Kause et al, 2004).

A major complication of reduced level of consciousness is the patient's ability to maintain a patent airway. While a patient with a reduced level of consciousness may appear to have a patent airway (i.e. they are unconscious but are breathing with ease), they may not have an effective or functioning cough or gag reflex. This means that the airway is *patent* but not *protected*. A patient who does not have an effective or functioning cough or gag reflex is in danger of aspirating stomach contents or retaining sputum, both of which can have fatal consequences. It is vital that nurses can recognise this potential life-threatening condition, get appropriate help immediately, and instigate immediate measures such as placing the patient in the recovery position and making sure that suction apparatus is to hand. Assessment and management of the patient's airway is discussed more fully in Chapter 4.

As well as evaluating the patient's level of consciousness to assess the status of the airway, it is also important to establish a baseline so that any improvement or deterioration of the patient's conscious level can be detected. As conscious level deteriorates, the patient's awareness and ability to adapt to their external environment also deteriorates. This may result in complications such as pressure sores, hypothermia and dehydration. As unconsciousness progresses, assimilation and adjustment to the internal environment deteriorates. Functions of the autonomic nervous

Box 7.1 Causes of impaired conscious level.
Reproduced from Ridley S, Smith G, Batchelor A, *Core Cases in Critical Care*, copyright 2002 with permission of Cambridge University Press.

Metabolic factors
- Cerebral anoxia/hypoxia
- Hypoglycaemia
- Thiamine deficiency and Wernicke's encephalopathy

Organ dysfunction
- Hyperglycaemia
- Respiratory failure
- Renal failure
- Hepatic failure
- Pancreatitis
- Hypopituitarism
- Adrenal dysfunction
- Thyroid dysfunction
- Sepsis
- Psychiatric disorders

Electrolyte and acid–base disturbances
- Hyper- and hyponatraemia
- Hyperosmolar conditions
- Hypercalcaemia
- Metabolic acidosis and alkalosis

Status epilepticus
- Focal or generalised fits

Drugs and toxins
- Alcohol
- Opiods
- Tricyclic antidepressants
- Carbon monoxide poisoning

Body temperature
- Hyper- and hypothermia

Intracranial pathology
- Stroke
- Intracranial haemorrhage
- Hydrocephalus
- Cerebral oedema
- Intracranial tumour, abscess or infection.

system become impaired and life-threatening situations can result where the patient loses control of vital responses such as breathing and circulation. Other complications of an impaired nervous system are the manifestation of fitting, or seizures, which can cause major complications, such as permanent brain damage or death (Wilkinson and Lennox, 2005). Types of coma are outlined in Box 7.2.

Box 7.2 Types of coma

Without focal signs or meningism – the most common form of coma generally resulting from anoxia, metabolic and toxic insults, infections and post-ictal states (Bateman, 2001).

With focal signs – damage of a particular area of the neuralgic system causing specific symptoms resulting from intracranial haemorrhage, infarction, tumour or abscess (Ginsberg, 1999).

With meningism – characterised by symptoms of irritability of the meninges, namely photophobia, irritability and headache (Ginsberg, 1999).

Without focal signs, but with meningism – associated with conditions such as subarachnoid haemorrhage, meningitis and meningo-encephalitis.

Key Point

Reduced consciousness can cause airway obstruction and death, and should be considered a medical emergency.

SECTION 2: NEUROLOGICAL ASSESSMENT

Due to the complexity of the nervous system, a full neurological assessment can take considerable time and skill. A comprehensive assessment will involve testing the following areas, working from the highest level of function to the lowest.

- Mental status and speech
- Cranial nerve function
- Motor function
- Sensory function
- Reflexes.

(Bickley and Hoekelman, 1999:569)

However, it is not necessary for the ward nurse to know, or be skilled in, all the components of a detailed neurological assessment, but s/he will need to be proficient in the initial neurological screen. This initial screen can be done in minutes, and the nurse can rapidly assess the extent of any neurological deficit in the patient, and evaluate to what extent this deficit might put the patient at risk. Finally, it is vital that the ward nurse knows when to get expert help in an emergency, or to call for a more comprehensive and skilled assessment.

For the nurse caring for the acutely ill adult patient, there are three main components in the rapid assessment of disability (D: neurological function) (Smith, 2003):

1. assessment of conscious level
2. pupil reaction
3. blood glucose levels.

During this rapid assessment, some components of cranial nerve and motor function are also incorporated.

1. Assessment of conscious level

Many clues to the patient's neurological status will have been picked up during the assessment of A, B and C (discussed in Chapters 4, 5 and 6). How the patient responds to you, what they say, and how they position themselves will all give clues as to their mental status and level of consciousness. In an emergency situation, it is easy to forget simple steps and leave out useful tests, so vital information is not to hand when summoning expert help. By using the simple steps of '**look**, **listen** and **feel**', and a systematic approach to the neurological assessment, your thoughts will be organised and everything pertinent will be covered.

The two common methods used to assess conscious level are: AVPU (Awake/Voice/Pain/Unresponsive) and GCS (the Glasgow Coma Scale). Both systems will be discussed in more detail.

Awake/Voice/Pain/Unresponsive (AVPU)
The AVPU scale (Box 7.3) is simple and quick to use, and can rapidly ascertain if the patient is at risk of airway obstruction.

Box 7.3 AVPU

A Is the patient **A**lert?
V Does the patient respond to your **V**oice
P Does the patient respond to **P**ain?
U Is the patient **U**nresponsive?

How to use AVPU

Look at the patient. Are they awake and alert, taking in their surroundings? If so they are **alert**.

Listen to them. Are they talking normally and making sense? If so, they are *orientated*.

A measure of orientation can be described as x 1, x 2 or x 3 and denotes whether the patient:

• Knows who they are
• Knows where they are
• Knows what date it is.

But remember, patients may have moved from ward to ward, and been unwell for a number of days, so a pragmatic approach may need to be taken. There is a marked difference in knowing you are in a hospital somewhere, and thinking you are at the airport!

If the patient has their eyes closed, talk to them to get a response. If the patient opens their eyes, they are responsive to **voice**. However, you need to note the difference between sleep, which is normal loss of consciousness, and abnormal loss of consciousness due to impairment of the neurological system (Wilkinson and Lennox, 2005).

Abnormal responses to voice can also be described as lethargic or stuporous. A lethargic patient appears sleepy, but needs to be stimulated to remain awake. A stuporous patient is difficult to arouse and may moan, withdraw or roll around during examination (Mangione, 2000).

 A stuporous patient may not respond to voice, but need shaking. If the patient does not respond to voice or gentle shaking, painful stimuli will need to be applied, and the level of response assessed. If there is a response, then the patient has responded to **pain**. The range of responses to pain can be extensive, ranging from the fairly high level localisation to the pain, to a more abnormal response seen in a generalised extensor reflex. Pain stimulus is discussed more fully later in this chapter.

If the patient makes no response, then they are **unresponsive**. Patients who only respond to pain or are unresponsive, or who are neurologically deteriorating, are at high risk of airway obstruction and will need to have their airway safeguarded and be referred urgently to critical care experts.

In a study of over 1300 patients who had been poisoned, it was reported that there was an association between AVPU scores and the Glasgow Coma Scale (Kelly et al, 2004):

A GCS 15
V GCS 12–14
P GCS 7–9
U GCS 3

Therefore patients with an AVPU of 'P' or 'U' could be regarded as being the equivalent GCS of < 9, and should therefore be considered to be at risk of obstructing their airway and should be further assessed by an anaesthetist.

The simple score of AVPU is useful as a rapid, easy technique for assessing conscious level but should not replace the more sophisticated Glasgow Coma Scale (GCS). If any reduction in level of consciousness is detected from the initial assessment, a GCS assessment should be performed by a skilled clinician.

Glasgow Coma Scale (GCS)

The most widely used assessment tool for evaluating conscious level is the Glasgow Coma Scale. A 14-point GCS was first published by Teasdale and Jennet in 1974, and was later developed into the currently used 15-point scale. The GCS provided consistency in the structure and terminology used in the assessment of conscious level in head injured patients. Although GCS is the gold standard for assessing conscious level and has worldwide application, it requires skill to achieve consistency in scoring (McNarry and Goldhill, 2004) and nurses find it more difficult to use than AVPU (Kelly et al, 2004).

The Glasgow Coma Scale is divided between the eye (E), verbal (V) and motor (M) responses of the patient. The patient who is fully awake and responsive will score 15/15, and the patient who is completely unresponsive will score 3/15. Documentation of GCS should include the overall GCS score, but it is also useful to break down the score into its separate components of eye opening (E), verbal response (V) and motor response (M). So, a patient who opens his eyes when you talk to him, moans and groans, and pushes you away when you apply painful stimuli will score 10/15 and should be recorded as E = 3, V = 2, M = 5. It is also good practice to provide a written description of the patient's precise responses as well as a numerical scale (Wilkinson and Lennox, 2005). The scale is shown in Box 7.4.

Eye opening   The patient should be observed before being stimulated to detect spontaneous eye opening. If the patient's eye are not open then speak to the patient; if they still remain closed after speaking, try gentle shaking, or the application of painful stimuli.

Eye opening indicates that the arousal mechanisms in the brain are active (Teasdale and Jennet, 1974). The arousal system

Box 7.4 The Glasgow Coma Scale

	Score	Response
Eye opening	4	Spontaneous
(E)	3	To speech
	2	To pain
	1	None
Verbal	5	Orientated conversation
response (V)	4	Confused speech
	3	Inappropriate words
	2	Incomprehensible sounds
	1	None
Motor	6	Obeys commands
response	5	Localises to pain
(M)	4	Withdraws from pain (normal flexion)
	3	Abnormal flexion
	2	Extension
	1	None

consists of the reticular activating system (RAS), which is part of the reticular formation, present throughout the brain stem extending into the diencephalon and spinal cord (Tortora and Grabowski, 2000). The RAS is activated through impulses such as noise, light and pain, and once activated stimulates the cerebral cortex causing arousal (Tortora and Grabowski, 2000). However, eye opening alone does not necessarily indicate awareness (Teasdale and Jennet, 1974). Cognitive function needs to be assessed to ensure that orientation, memory, attention and registration are intact (Talley and O'Connor, 2001).

Problems may arise with assessing eye opening if the patient's eyes are swollen shut due to trauma. If this is the case, a 'C' should be recorded on the assessment chart to show that the patient's eyes were Closed and eye opening could not be assessed.

Verbal response The ability to use language is one of the highest functions of the human brain (Mangione, 2000), and involves several complex activities that include sensory and motor areas of the cortex. The speech centre is located in Broca's area in the left frontal lobe in 97% of the population (Tortora and Grabowski, 2000). Damage to speech areas in the brain can cause different manifestations of speech disorder, or aphasia. Articulation of speech also involves the complex manipulation of the larynx, vocal cords, face, tongue and lips (Tortora and Grabowski, 2000). Speech also indicates that the patient has an intact airway.

If the patient has an endotracheal tube or tracheostomy in place, they will not be able give a verbal response and a 'T' should be recorded on the assessment chart to indicate the patient had a tracheal Tube in situ.

Motor response   As well as assessing the motor response separately, it is useful to note the patient's responses while assessing eye opening and verbal responses. At a high level of motor function, the patient should be able to *obey simple commands*, such as poking out their tongue or touching their nose. The command to squeeze fingers should be avoided, as the presence of the fingers in the patient's palm may stimulate the automatic grasp reflex (Teasdale and Jennet, 1974).

If the patient does not respond to commands, painful stimuli should be applied and a range of responses will be observed. The pain response tests the thalamus function at the uppermost level of the brain stem (Mangione, 2000). The proper response is to push away the painful stimulus, which indicates that the patient is *localising to pain*. Teasdale and Jennet (1974) advise testing localisation to pain in more than one place. An improper response is to assume a certain posture. The reaction to painful stimuli is discussed more fully later in the chapter.

Abnormal flexion indicates mild thalamic dysfunction and is also termed decorticate posturing. The patient holds the upper arms close to their sides with their elbows, wrists and fingers flexed. The legs are internally rotated and extended, with plantars (feet) flexed (Bickley and Hoekelman, 1999).

Extension is seen in severe thalamic dysfunction, and termed decerebrate posturing. The arms are adducted and extended at the elbows, forearms pronated, wrists and fingers flexed. The legs are extended at the knees, with plantars flexed. This posture indicates a lesion in the diencephalon, which includes the thalamus, the midbrain or pons, but may be a result of severe metabolic disorders such as hypoxia, or hypoglycaemia (Bickley and Hoekelman, 1999).

No motor response to painful stimuli indicates the thalamus is entirely dysfunctional. There may be a bending of the knees, but this is a simple spinal reflex (Mangione, 2000). When there is no response, spinal transection should be considered and excluded (Teasdale and Jennet 1974).

It is important that conscious level is assessed only after A, B and C have been assessed and treated. Levels of consciousness can be affected by initial problems with the airway, breathing and circulation, and these should be ruled out. Assessing patient responses can also be complicated if the patient has suffered a spinal injury, causing paralysis. Although it might be a rare presentation in the general ward patient, care should be taken with any patient who has a history that might lead you to suspect a spinal injury, such as a fall. If you suspect the patient has a spinal injury, the patient should be immobilised with a neck collar and spinal board until the spine can be medically cleared.

Key Point

If the patient has had a history of a fall that may have resulted in a neck injury, always consider spinal injury and take precautions until proven otherwise.

Painful stimuli

There are a number of ways to elicit a painful stimulus to assess the patient's response. While it is a necessary intervention, the practitioner should aim to determine the patient's response as quickly as possible while causing minimal tissue damage (Guin, 1997). The application of the stimulus should start with the least noxious, such as talking to the patient and shaking them, before moving on to inflicting pain.

The most common methods of painful stimuli are:

- Nail bed compression
- Supra orbital pressure
- Sternal rub
- Trapezium squeeze
- Earlobe pressure

There is debate whether painful stimulus should be applied centrally or peripherally, the argument being that peripheral stimuli such as nail bed pressure might result in a spinal response. For that reason painful stimuli should not be applied to the legs. Each type of painful stimulus has its advantages and disadvantages and may not be practical in patients with specific injuries, such as orbital swelling. The sternal rub appears to be the most commonly applied stimulus as it is the easiest area to access, but repeated application of the stimulus may cause extensive bruising and be distressing to relatives. The chest area is also a useful place to test capillary refill time (CRT) (see Chapter 4) and bruising may cause problems with this assessment. The trapezium squeeze involves squeezing the large muscle between the neck and the shoulder. There is no published evidence as to the best painful stimulus to use, but the trapezium squeeze seems the most practical; as well as being an effective source of pain, it can appear less aggressive to any relatives present.

2. Pupil reaction

The pupil in the eye should be inspected for size, shape and symmetry (Bickley and Hoekelman, 1999). The size of the pupil should be measured in millimetres, the normal range in size being between 2 and 6 mm (Sheppard and Wright, 2003). A light is shone into the eye from the side to test the pupillary reflex. This tests the function of the midbrain (Mangione, 2000) and the cranial nerves II and III, and the optic nerve and oculomotor nerve. The normal pupillary response to light is to constrict briskly and equally in both eyes.

Drug therapy that may affect pupils' reaction include opioids and muscarinic agonists (pilocarpine, bethanechol) that constrict the pupil, and muscarinic anatagonists (atropine, hyoscine) that dilate the pupil (Rang et al, 1999). As well as checking the patient's drug prescriptions, it is also important to know of any previous ocular injury or congenital abnormality that may affect the evaluation of the pupillary response (Bateman, 2001). If the patient is unable to tell you their history, relatives may have the information.

3. Blood glucose levels

Any patient with an altered level of consciousness should have their blood glucose levels checked at the bedside to rule out hypoglycaemia and hyperglycaemia. Normal blood glucose levels are between 4 and 8 mmol/l. Low blood glucose or hypoglycaemia is the most common presentation, and can occur in hospitalised patients with no history of diabetes. Symptoms of hunger, dizziness and confusion can occur at blood glucose levels of less than 2.2 mmol/l (40 mg/100 ml) (Laycock and Wise, 1996), and if untreated can lead to coma and death. High blood glucose levels (hyperglycaemia) are more common among diabetic patients and will present with other metabolic disturbances such as hypokalaemia and dehydration. Treatment of blood glucose disturbances will be discussed later in this chapter and those associated with sepsis have been discussed in Chapter 6.

In the deteriorating ward patient, blood glucose levels can be rapidly assessed, and either ruled out or treated, before more advanced assessments or investigations are organised.

Key Point

Do your A–B–C–D–E, but don't forget **D, E, F, G – Don't Ever Forget Glucose!**

INVESTIGATIONS AND THE INITIAL TREATMENT OF THE NEUROLOGICALLY COMPROMISED PATIENT

Investigating the patient with reduced level of consciousness

It is essential that a patient with a reduced level of consciousness is assessed by an expert. A history should be taken and a physical examination undertaken before any additional more complex investigations are ordered. As a matter of course, blood tests for urea and electrolytes, blood glucose, full blood count, clotting and arterial blood gases may already have been considered during the A, B and C phase of the assessment, as would chest x-ray. However, a number of other investigations may also be considered such as computerised tomographic (CT) scanning, magnetic resonance imaging (MRI) and lumbar puncture.

- *Computerised tomographic (CT) scanning*   CT scanning can be used to investigate intracranial lesions and the spine. Horizontal x-ray images are taken of the body to detect areas of different levels of density, and whether these have caused anatomical alterations in the normal structures.
- *Magnetic resonance imaging (MRI)*   MRI is a more recent advance than CT scanning and uses magnetic pulses to relay information about the physical properties of the tissue. Images can be reconstructed to give views in any plane with greater ease and resolution than possible with a CT scan (Ginsberg, 1999). Both MRI and CT scan images can be further enhanced by using contrast mediums.
- *Lumbar puncture*   A lumbar puncture is performed to obtain specimens of cerebrospinal fluid to commonly analyse for infection (bacterial, viral and fungal) and cytology. Contra-indications to lumbar puncture are: suspected intracranial mass, where there is a risk of herniation of the brain through the tentorium or foramen magnum, causing fatal compression of the brain stem; local infection; bleeding disorders or significant spinal deformity (Ginsberg, 1999).

Both CT scanning and MRI necessitate the patient being transferred to the x-ray department and consideration needs to be given to the safety of the patient during transfer and the prevention of further deterioration. Expert help should be sought to assist with the transfer and an anaesthetist may be required to manage the airway. Care of the acutely unwell patient being transferred is discussed in the Chapter 9.

A lumbar puncture can be performed at the bedside, but there needs to be cooperation from the patient in order to be successful in this delicate manoeuvre. Confused and agitated patients may need sedating and, again, the anaesthetist may be needed to provide safe care during the procedure.

> **Key Point**
>
> Always ensure the patient has been physiologically optimised, is adequately monitored, and that you have skilled clinicians before you transfer an acutely unwell patient (see Chapter 9).

Patients who have reduced level of consciousness, new onset muscle weakness or impaired sensation may have problems swallowing. Swallowing is a complex process involving the proper functioning of six cranial nerves and involves both voluntary and involuntary and reflex muscle action (Iggulden, 2006). The cough and gag reflex are an integral part of an effective swallow and impairment or absence of these reflexes means the patient does not have a protected airway and is at risk of airway obstruction and aspiration. If there are any concerns with the patient's ability to effectively swallow, the patient should be made 'nil by mouth' until a competent practitioner can perform a swallow assessment.

Signs that a patient may not have an effective swallow include:

- Their medical history and diagnosis
- Coughing and choking
- Drooling
- Breathlessness and oxygen desaturation
- 'Wet' voice.

Any patient with suspected impaired swallowing is in danger of aspirating food and drink into their lungs, resulting in pneumonia, which could lead to death. A nasogastric tube can be inserted in order that the patient can receive adequate nutrition and hydration.

Treating the causes of reduced levels of consciousness

Once A, B and C have been assessed and treated, the patient's conscious level (D) may have improved with oxygen, assisted ventilation and fluids. If the patient still has a reduced level of consciousness, there are a number of measures that can be taken that may prevent further deterioration.

Seizures

Seizures can occur in acutely unwell ward patients for a variety of reasons such as infection, metabolic disturbances and hypoxia, as well as in patients who have been diagnosed as epileptic.

Seizures are a result of abnormal electrical discharges in the brain causing sudden unconsciousness and violent uncontrolled body movement (Wilkinson and Lennox, 2005). Of the two main types of seizures – primary generalised and focal – it is the primary generalised tonic-clonic seizure that is the most likely presentation in the acutely ill ward patient. Characterised by loss of consciousness and random disorganised body jerking, these types of seizures can cause hypoxia and acidosis if prolonged or untreated. Status epilepticus is the occurrence of one tonic-clonic seizure after another without recovery of consciousness between attacks. If the seizures go on for more than 1 hour, there is a risk of permanent brain damage (Wilkinson and Lennox, 2005).

Management of seizures involves protecting the airway, preventing limb injury and awaiting recovery. Records should be made describing the frequency and appearance of the seizure, and expert help should be sought. If attacks are frequent then intravenous diazepam or lorazepam should be considered as well as the patient's normal epilepsy medication. If seizures do not respond to first-line drugs, then phenytoin or phenobarbitone should be considered, and anaesthesia with thiopentone might be a necessity.

Key Point

Patients who have seizures can have very poor outcomes: always seek help.

Hypo- and hyperglycaemia

Altered level of consciousness due to high blood glucose can be treated with 50 units of Actrapid or Humulin S insulin in 49 ml

0.9% saline via syringe driver. The rate of infusion will depend on the extent of the hyperglycaemia, but can be 4 ml/hr for a blood glucose of > 8 mmol/l or 6 ml/hr if the blood glucose is > 11 mmol/l. Fluid and potassium levels will also need to be monitored and replaced.

Patients with low blood glucose will need their blood sugar levels increasing with approximately 10–20 g of glucose. This can be provided by two teaspoons of sugar, three sugar lumps or a sugary drink such as a cola or Lucozade. Ensure that the patient can safely swallow. For a semi-conscious or uncooperative patient, *GlucoGel*® (formerly known as *Hypostop Gel*® glucose 9.2 g/23-g oral ampoule) can be rubbed onto the mucous membranes. These measures can be be repeated every 10–15 minutes. For unconscious patients, 50 ml of 20% glucose can be given via infusion into a large vein (British National Formulary 54).

Drug overdose and poisoning

Although the patient presenting with overdose and poisoning is more commonly associated with accident and emergency care, the general ward patient can also present with symptoms of drug overdose and poisoning. Some of the agents responsible may have been prescribed as part of the patient's treatment, such as opiates or benzodiazepines, but it is not unknown for patients to take recreational drugs bought in by relatives. Many of the substances involved in poisoning and overdose can produce similar signs and symptoms. Immediate management involves supporting the patient's vital signs as well as treating the underlying cause.

For more comprehensive information regarding the treatment of patients who have had an overdose, the National Poisons Information Service at www.npis.org and TOXBASE® at www.toxbase.co.uk are both useful resources available on the Internet.

- *Opioid overdose* causing reduced level of consciousness may be suspected from the patient's history, prescription charts and pinpoint pupils. Intravenous naloxone 0.4–2 mg can be given and repeated at 2 to 3 minute intervals, up to a maximum of 10 mg. If respiratory function does not improve, reassess the diagnosis (British National Formulary 54). Any opioid infusions should be stopped and alternative pain relief prepared.

* *Benzodiazepine* overdose, such as midazolam, can happen after procedures and the antidote flumazenil can be given by intravenous injection: 200 micrograms over 15 seconds.

Suspected stroke

Stroke is a condition that involves any disease process that disrupts blood flow to a focal region of the brain. Clinical presentation depends on the area of the brain affected and can involve limb weakness and numbness, speech and swallowing problems or coma and death (Ma, Cline et al, 2004). Stroke can affect the individual at any time and is not an uncommon complication in the acute adult hospital patient. Stroke should be suspected in any patient who has rapidly developing signs of focal or global disturbance of cerebral function.

Diagnosis can be established through careful history taking, examination and investigation. A CT scan is recommended within 24 hours of the onset of symptoms, followed by considering MRI if the diagnosis is in doubt (Royal College of Physicians, 2004). Stroke is a medical emergency and the patient needs to be closely monitored to prevent further complications, such as aspiration and airway problems.

Head injury

Patients who present to the accident and emerergency (A&E) department with a head injury may be admitted to a general ward for observation for a number of reasons, and it may not be uncommon for patients with moratley severe head injuries to be admitted to District General Hospitals. The National Institute for Health and Clinical Excellence (NICE, 2007) guidance on the management of head injuries clearly states the care and management of the patient in A&E and recommends admission to hospital if the following criteria are met:

* New, clinically significant abnormalities on imaging
* Not returned to GCS of 15 after imaging (regardless of imaging results)
* Delay in CT scan

- Persistent vomiting or severe headaches
- Drug or alcohol intoxication, other injuries, shock, suspected non-accidental injury, meningism, cerebrospinal fluid leak.

The patient should be admitted, under the care of a consultant trained in head injury management, to an area where nurses caring for the patient are competent in assessing vital signs (temperature, pulse, respiratory rate, blood pressure and oxygen saturation) and the Glasgow Coma Scale. NICE (2007) guidance recommends half-hourly observations until the GCS is 15. Senior medical assessment and further CT scanning should be considered if the patient's condition changes and displays any of the following:

- New agitation or abnormal behaviour
- GCS dropping by 1 point for 30 minutes
- Any drop of 3 or more points in eye opening or verbal response, or 2 or more in motor response score
- Severe or increasing headache or persistent vomiting
- New or evolving neurological symptoms, such as pupil inequality or asymmetry of limb or facial movement.

(NICE, 2007)

Nursing management of patient with reduced consciousness

Managing a patient with a reduced level of consciousness involves the continual assessment of A, B, C and D.

- **A** Maintaining an airway, using manual procedures such as head tilt, chin lift, or jaw thrust if necessary. Adjuncts such as a Guedel or nasopharyngeal airway might be necessary. For patients with a GCS of < 9, the patient should be reviewed by an anaesthetist because endotracheal intubation may be necessary. Nursing the patient in the recovery position may help to keep the airway patent, but it may not prevent aspiration of stomach contents and suction apparatus to clear secretions should be available. Keep nil by mouth if the patient has a reduced level of consciousness or you suspect the swallow is ineffective.

- **B** Maintain adequate oxygenation using 10–15l oxygen via non-rebreathe mask, or assist breathing using a bag valve mask. Adequate air entry should be assessed using auscultation with a stethoscope. Arterial blood gases will give important information on effectiveness of breathing as well as information about the metabolic state of the patient (pH, base excess and lactate).
- **C** Maintain adequate circulation with intravenous fluid, but avoid aggressive re-hydration if raised intracranial pressure is suspected. Monitor urine output and catheterise if necessary. Maintain a normal body temperature by using warming or cooling equipment if necessary.
- **D** Record neurological observations every 15–30 minutes. These should include vital signs (temperature, pulse, blood pressure, respiratory rate and oxygen saturations) as well as pupil reaction and Glasgow Coma Scale (GCS). Monitor and record any seizures. Patients who complain of sudden onset headaches, or have headaches associated with nausea, photophobia and neck stiffness should be more fully assessed. Blood pressure should be monitored and pain relief given.

Other considerations are to prevent pressure damage and maintain basic hygiene cares, such as cleanliness and mouth and eye care.

SUMMARY OF CHAPTER

This chapter has reviewed the assessment and initial treatment measures for the disability (D) section of the A–B–C–D–E assessment model. This brief overview of the neurological system, its anatomy and physiology and the neurological disorders common to the acutely ill ward patient have provided a knowledge base for the nurse to begin to develop his/her assessment skills. By practising neurological assessment skills; AVPU and GCS, the nurses will become adept at recognising and managing the neurologically impaired acutely ill ward patient. The nurse can test his/her knowledge by going through the case scenarios at the end of this chapter. Skills will be honed by practising these assessment techniques in real-life situations.

CHAPTER 7: SCENARIOS

Scenario 7.1

Mrs M, a 69-year-old retired teacher has returned to the ward from recovery, following an endoscopic retrograde cholangio-pancreatography (ERCP). Her first set of observations on return to the ward were: airway patent and protected (able to cough), respiratory rate (RR) 18/min, SpO$_2$ 98% on air, BP 120/76, pulse 72 regular, has not yet passed urine, rousable with gentle shaking, appears orientated.

After 45 minutes, the Health Care Assistant informs you that she can't wake the patient up.

Q 1 What would you do next?

When you assess Mrs M, she is snoring loudly and is only responding to pain.

Q 2 What are your actions?

Q 3 What further information might the medical or outreach teams need?

Q 4 How can you further treat Mrs M?

Answers to scenario 7.1

Q1 You need to assess A–B–C–D–E. Ensure you can wake Mrs M and that she has an adequate airway.

Q2 Use manual manoeuvres (head tilt/chin lift) or adjuncts (nasopharyngeal or oral pharyngeal airway) to maintain the airway. Apply high-flow oxygen via a non-rebreathe facemask. Ensure there is adequate venous access. Call urgently for the patient's medical team and contact critical care if the GCS is less than 9.

Q3 They will want to know the patient's blood glucose levels and pupil reaction as well as what sedation the patient was given

Q4 If the patient was given a benzodiazepine such as mida-zolam, she may benefit from the antidote flumazenil by intravenous injection, 200 micrograms over 15 seconds. Abnormal blood sugar should be treated with glucose or insulin.

Scenario 7.2

Mr C, a 41-year-old cab driver was admitted to the ward area from A&E after taking approximately 100 Venlafaxine (37.5mg). He has had a history of depression for two years.

On admission to A&E, his assessment was as follows: airway patent and protected, SpO_2 98% on air, RR 18, BP 135/95, pulse 92 and regular, GCS 15/15, orientated x 3.

When he got to the ward he had a two seizures, which resolved spontaneously. His GCS is 15/15, PERL, BM 3.8mmol/l.

Q 1   What would you do next?

You're not sure about the drugs he has taken.

Q 2   How can you find out more about the side effects so you can monitor him adequately?

Q 3   You've found out about the effects of Venlafaxine; how are you going to monitor Mr C?

Mr C does not seem to be improving and is not waking up between seizures.

Q 4   What will you do next?

Answers to case study 7.2

Q1 You need to assess A–B–C–D–E and refer the patient to his medical team with information about the seizures.

Q2 You can contact the National Poisons Information Service at www.npis.org and use TOXBASE® for information about the drugs that Mr C took. This can be done online or by phone.

Q3 He needs a 12-lead ECG to detect arrhythmias associated with the drug. Prepare PR or IV diazepam in case he has another seizure. Monitor oxygen saturation (SpO_2) and give oxygen if SpO_2 is less than 94%. Monitor blood glucose levels. Prepare to take arterial blood gases if SpO$_2$ drops further and call critical care if SpO$_2$ goes below 90%, seizures continue, conscious level deteriorates, or you are concerned.

Q4 If Mr C continues to deteriorate or have seizures, you need to refer him to critical care. He may need more potent drugs to control his seizures and you should consider transferring him to a higher level of care.

Scenario 7.3

Ben is 19 years old and while he was in hospital following an appendicectomy he has been visited by his friends. After visiting time you notice that Ben looks a bit pale and is lying on his bed asleep. When you assess him he has a patent airway, but is not responding to you. His BP is 90/45 and his pupils are pinpoint.

Q 1 What would you do next?

While you are waiting for help to arrive, you notice that Ben looks a bit grey and his breathing is very shallow.

Q 2 What should you do?

Answers to scenario 7.3

Q1 You need to call for urgent help. Put Ben in the recovery position and ensure he has a patent airway. Give him high-flow oxygen via a non-rebreathe mask. Make sure you have working suction to hand in case he vomits. You need to get venous access and start fluids. Prepare naloxone 0.4–2 mg.

Q2 Put out a cardiac arrest call. Lay him on his back and start the Basic Life Support algorithm. If he has an output, supplement his breathing by using a bag, valve mask with high-flow oxygen.

Scenario 7.4

Mrs D is a diabetic who has come into hospital to be treated for a septic leg ulcer. When you go to do her leg dressing, you notice she feels a bit clammy and she is not fully responsive.

Q 1 What would you do next?

Her blood pressure is 90/45 and heart rate 115 bpm. You notice her fingers and toes feel quite cold and her central temperature is only 34.9 °C.

Q 2 What other information might be useful?

Q 3 What should you do next?

Answers to scenario 7.4

Q1 You need to assess A–B–C–D–E

Q2 She is showing signs of sepsis and a blood culture should be taken. Arterial blood gases should also be assessed for metabolic acidosis.

Q3 Call her medical team and critical care outreach.

Apply high-flow oxygen and prepare to give fluids such as normal saline or gelofusine.

Keep her warm and monitor closely.

REFERENCES

Bateman DE (2001) Neurological Assessment of Coma. Journal of Neurology, Neurosurgery and Psychiatry 71:113–117

Bickley LS, Hoekelman RA (1999) Bate's Guide to Physical Examination and History Taking. Lippincott, Philadelphia

British National Formulary 54. http://bnf.org/bnf/bnf/current/4195.htm

Buist M, Bernard S, et al (2004) Association between clinically abnormal observations and subsequent in-hospital mortality: a prospective study. Resuscitation 62(2):137–141

Ginsberg L (1999) Neurology (7th edn). Blackwell Science. Oxford

Guin PR (1997) Eye opening, verbal and motor response to three types of painful stimuli (nail bed pressure, sternal rub and trapezial grip) in patients with impaired consciousness. PhD thesis. University of Florida

Iggulden H (2006) Care of the Neurological Patient. Blackwell Publishing, Oxford

Kause J, Smith G, et al (2004) A comparison of antecedents to cardiac arrests, deaths and emergency intensive care admissions in Australia and New Zealand, and the United Kingdom – the ACADEMIA study. Resuscitation 62:275–282

Kelly CA, Upex A, Bateman DN (2004) Comparison of consciousness level assessment in the poisoned patient using the Alert/Verbal/Painful/Unresponsive Scale and Glasgow Coma Scale. Annals of Emergency Medicine 44(2):108–113

Laycock J, Wise P (1996) Essential Endocrinology (3rd edn). Oxford University Press. Oxford

Ma OJ, Cline DM, Tintinalli JE, Kelen GD, Stapczynski JS (2004) Emergency Medicine (2nd edn). McGraw-Hill, New York.

Mangione S (2000) Physical Diagnosis Secrets. Hanley and Belfus, Inc. Philadelphia

McNarry AF, Goldhill DR (2004) Simple bedside assessment of level of consciousness: comparison of two simple assessment scales with the Glasgow Coma Scale. Anaesthesia 59(1):34–37

NICE (2007) Head Injury. National Institute for Health and Clinical Excellence, London

Rang HP, Dale MM, Ritter JM (1999) Pharmacology (4th edn). Churchill Livingstone, London

Ridley S, Smith G, Batchelor A (2002) Core Cases in Critical Care. Greenwich Medical Media, London.

Royal College of Physicians (2004) National Clinical Guidelines for Stroke. Intercollegiate Stroke Working Party, Royal College of Physicians, London

Schein RM, Hazday HN, et al (1990) Clinical antecedents to in-hospital cardiopulmonary arrest. Chest 98(6):1338–1392

Sheppard M, Wright M (2003) High Dependency Nursing. Bailliere Tindall, London

Smith G (2003) ALERT. Acute Life Threatening Events Rocognition and Treatment. University of Portsmouth

Talley NJ, O'Connor S (2001). Clinical Examination (4th edn). Blackwell Science, Oxford

Teasdale G, Jennett B (1974) Assessment of coma and impaired consciousness. The Lancet 2(7872) July 13: 81–83

Tortora GJ, Grabowski SR (2000) Principles of Anatomy and Physiology (9th edn). John Wiley & Sons, New York

Wilkinson I, Lennox G (2005) Essential Neurology (4th edn). Blackwell Publishing, Oxford

A–B–C–D–**E**: Everything that Should Be Considered for Other Potential Problems

8

INTRODUCTION

Although the focus of rapid assessment will always be the factors that are likely to kill the patient immediately (i.e. Airway, Breathing, Circulation), there are a number of other high-risk contributory factors which, if not recognised and treated, will become rapidly life-threatening.

Having carried out assessment of the patient's airway, breathing and circulation, with management of immediate problems, a further assessment of the patient as a whole should constitute an initial fast overview, exposing the limbs, abdomen and any foci of pain or discomfort. Care should be taken to ensure that the patient's dignity is maintained at all times.

LEARNING OBJECTIVES

At the end of this chapter you should be able to:

❏ List other important signs of potential acute problems identified by inspection, palpation and communication
❏ Describe the information that can be obtained from other sources such as charts, patient records, and diagnostic investigations
❏ Understand the abnormal markers of electrolyte and renal dysfunction
❏ List the inflammatory markers associated with infection and the inflammatory response.

FURTHER ASSESSMENT OF THE PATIENT

This should constitute a visual, palpatory and auscultatory overview, including the following.

 Look for:

- Signs of inflammation (reddening, swelling, induration)
- Signs of ischaemia (purple/black necrotic areas or limbs)
- Signs of haemorrhage (obvious blood loss, loss into wound drains, swelling in soft tissues, melaena or haematemesis)
- Signs of allergy or anaphylaxis (flushing, or a skin rash may be visible)
- Signs of bruising or haemorrhagic rashes.

 Listen to:

- Any complaints of pain from the patient. (All of the above will produce local pain and it is important to ask the patient where the pain is, if they have any)
- The patient and his/her family for the background and context of the problem.

 Feel for:

- Obvious swelling and distension (pay particular attention to the abdomen)
- Calf pain (unilateral may be a deep vein thrombosis)
- Surgical emphysema (air in the subcutaneous tissues), which can develop from a leak through the pleura.

Providing that nothing immediately requires a response you should go on to a more detailed assessment using information from other sources. These include charts, notes, laboratory investigations, scans and x-rays and other members of the multidisciplinary team as well as the patient's family.

Charts

Observation charts

The last week or so of observation charts should be reviewed to detect any trends in temperature, HR, BP, RR, SpO_2. HR often rises with temperature and if there is sepsis, blood pressure may also fall. Level of consciousness should be recorded with every observation of the patient (see Chapter 7).

An increased temperature will be associated with increased sweating and fluid loss from respiration (known as insensible loss) – the normal is about 500 ml/24 hours, which is increased by 13% for every 1 °C rise in temperature. Thus a patient with a 40 °C temperature will lose approx 200 ml/day extra from this alone.

Neurological observation and pain charts

Look for any ongoing trends such as a steadily rising blood pressure and tachycardia on the neurological chart, or an increasing pain score unrelieved by analgesia on the pain chart.

Fluid balance charts

Fluid balance charts should also be viewed over the previous 2–3 days to understand the full picture of the patient's fluid status. Look for extra fluid losses such as vomiting, watery diarrhoea, and ileostomy losses. Any fluid losses from the GI tract should alert a review of electrolytes, particularly sodium and potassium, which are lost from the GI tract. Increased respiratory rate and mouth breathing will increase insensible fluid losses, particularly if the patient is inhaling dry oxygen. Whenever possible, humidified oxygen should be provided if the patient is likely to be on it for more than 6 hours.

Don't forget to review the previous 2–3 days' blood glucose measurements if they are being done as well. Look for changes associated with similar times of the day (for instance, are they getting their insulin too early and dropping blood glucose levels?).

Note: Remember to check the mathematics – fluid balance charts are notoriously inaccurate.

Prescription charts

A review of the patient's regular and PRN drugs will give more information about underlying causes, and intravenous fluids. In addition, consider whether side effects or direct effects from one of the drugs might be contributing in some way to the patient's problems: for instance, if the patient has been receiving beta blockers and has a low blood pressure or heart rate. Or if a new drug has recently been prescribed and given, it is possible that the patient may have had a reaction to it.

Laboratory investigations

Electrolytes

Abnormalities in one electrolyte level are often associated with other electrolyte alterations and it is worth reviewing all the significant electrolyte levels to ensure that nothing is missed. These include sodium, potassium, magnesium, calcium, phosphate and chloride. Abnormalities are commonly associated with fluid volume changes in intravascular, extracellular and intracellular spaces.

An assessment of fluid status of the patient (see Chapter 6) is essential both to diagnose and treat hypovolaemia but also in order to understand the cause of the problem. If the patient's levels are outside the normal range (see Table 8.1), make sure that the doctor is aware of this so that the appropriate treatment can be started.

Sodium can indicate the relative water state of the body. Low sodium levels can be caused by excess fluid, internal fluid shifts with sodium from the extracellular space or loss of sodium through use of diuretics or renal disease.

Table 8.1 Normal ranges for electrolytes

Electrolyte	Normal levels
Sodium	135–150 mmol/l
Potassium	3.5–5.0 mmol/l
Magnesium	0.75–1.05 mmol/l
Calcium (total)	2.12–2.65 mmol/l
Phosphate	0.8–1.45 mmol/l
Chloride	95–105 mmol/l

Note: Always check local laboratory reference ranges as these can vary

Hyponatremia (plasma sodium levels < 130 mmol/l)
Moderate hyponatremia commonly occurs as a side effect of thiazide diuretics (e.g. bendrofluazide), but other more severe causes include endocrine disorders and cardiac, liver or renal disease.

The patient may be asymptomatic at moderate levels (120–120 mmol/l) but below this they will be restless, confused and irritable, with seizures and coma occurring at sodium levels of less than 120 mmol/l.

Management should focus on maintaining intravascular and extracellular fluid volume and slow correction of the sodium levels, aiming at between 125 and 130 mmol/l at a rate of change of less than 20 mmol/l/day.

- *Decreased sodium levels with decreased extracellular fluid volume (body water and sodium loss).* This can be caused by osmotic diuresis, gastrointestinal losses, burns, pancreatitis and renal tubular disease.
  Fluid should be replaced with 0.9% sodium chloride, which will allow for both sodium and fluid volume replacement.
- *Decreased sodium levels with normal or excess extracellular fluid volume.* This can be caused by nephrotic syndrome, inappropriate anti-diuretic hormone secretion, water intoxication (e.g. TURP syndrome), drugs such as carbemazepine, etc.
  Fluid intake should be restricted to 1–1.5 l/day and if there are symptoms with oedema then furosemide may be used to increase diuresis with replacement of sodium using hypertonic

saline. This is usually done in intensive or high-dependency care so that frequent monitoring can be carried out.

Hypernatremia (plasma sodium levels > 150 mmol/l)
Hypernatremia can occur as a consequence of dehydration (the very young and the very old are particularly at risk) but is also associated with other causes such as diabetes insipidus and lithium toxicity.

The patient will be thirsty (unless there is central nervous system disease) at about 3–4 mmol/l above normal sodium levels. Lethargy, seizures, muscle tremor and coma are also associated with hypernatremia.

If these features are found during assessment then a recent blood sodium level is essential to rule out altered sodium levels. A urinary sodium level will also be useful to understand the cause.

The management of hypernatremia will depend on the cause and the speed with which the hypernatraemia has occurred. However, generally it is best to slowly correct the sodium level over 2–3 days to avoid sudden fluid shifts, which may cause cerebral oedema.

- *Increased sodium with decreased extracellular volume (excess body water loss with some sodium loss).* This can be caused by renal dysfunction, osmotic diuresis (e.g. that associated with diabetes mellitus), diabetes insipidus or excess sweating or GI losses. This is corrected by treating the cause (e.g. desmopressin for diabetes insipidus) and giving fluid – initially 0.9% sodium chloride but as the sodium level normalises this can switch to 5% glucose.
- *Increased sodium with normal extracellular volume (sodium is being retained or extra sodium has been given to the patient and there is no change in body water).* This can be caused by endocrine disorder such as Cushing's syndrome, or infusion of excess sodium bicarbonate or chloride.

Hypokalaemia (potassium level < 3.5 mmol/l)
Potassium is an essential intracellular electrolyte and the amount seen in the plasma is very small (approx. 1% of total body

potassium) by comparison. However, changes in the plasma level usually indicate movement of potassium into and out of the cells. Potassium levels often vary with hydrogen ion concentration as the two ions compete to move across cell membranes. In metabolic alkalosis, the hydrogen ion concentration in the renal tubules or in extracellular fluid is low; thus more potassium ions will be either excreted into the urine or transported into the cell and plasma potassium levels will fall. This is a cause of hypokalaemia. Low levels of potassium can increase the likelihood of arrhythmias, particularly if the patient is acutely unwell.

The symptoms of hypokalaemia are arrhythmias, constipation, weakness and ileus. The causes are usually either:

- Increased losses of potassium through gastrointestinal losses (diarrhoea, vomiting, fistula losses), or renal losses (diabetic ketoacidosis, renal tubular disease, endocrine disorders, diuretics); or
- Increased movement of potassium into the cells, as occurs in high glucose levels, and insulin treatment, acute alkalosis etc.

In terms of management, replacement of potassium is the treatment and the method will depend on the acuity of the symptoms and the level of potassium. If there are arrhythmias, then intravenous potassium (20 mmols infused over 30 minutes to 1 hour through a large or central vein) should be given. If there are no symptoms and the level is not too deranged then oral supplements can be given.

Hyperkalaemia (> 6.0 mmol/l)
Excretion of potassium levels is usually controlled by the kidneys but as most of the body's potassium is within the cells, anything that increases potassium release from the cells (e.g. rhabdomyolysis, drugs such as suxamethonium, metabolic acidosis) will also cause high potassium levels.

Symptoms include cardiac arrhythmias, including cardiac arrest, paresthesiae and weakness. Symptoms are related to the rate of the rise of potassium levels as well as the absolute levels.

ECG changes are associated with hyperkalaemia on a 12-lead ECG (tall or peaked T waves, flat P waves and extended PR interval).

Causes are:

- Reduced renal excretion, as in chronic renal failure, adrenal insufficiency, diabetes, use of potassium-sparing diuretics
- Increased release from cells occurs with acidosis, rhabdomyolysis, tumour lysis syndrome
- Iatrogenic – over-supplementation of potassium.

Management depends on treatment of the underlying cause. However, if arrhythmias or ECG changes are evident then 10–12 iu of insulin in 50 ml of 50% glucose should be infused over 20 minutes. Calcium supplements or resonium can be given. If the potassium level is > 7 mmol/l, then 10 ml of 10% calcium chloride should be given intravenously to stabilise the myocardial membrane.

Hypocalcaemia

Calcium is an essential component of muscle contraction and nerve conduction.

Symptoms of calcium deficiency range from paresthesiae and hyperreflexia to tetany, arrhythmias and seizures. Total calcium levels include 40% of calcium bound to albumin so only about 60% will be ionised calcium and active.

Causes of hypocalcaemia include renal failure, rhabdomyolysis, hypoparathyroidism, pancreatitis, osteomalacia, and critical illness.

Management can be effected by calcium supplementation, given intravenously in the acute situation with 10 ml of 10% calcium gluconate.

Hypercalcaemia

Once total plasma levels are > 3.5 mmol/l, then symptoms become apparent, although this will depend on the patient.

Symptoms include nausea, vomiting, muscle weakness, depression, coma, polyuria, renal calculi, renal failure, renal stones and polydipsia. Ultimately cardiac arrest can occur.

Causes are most commonly malignancy, particularly bone metasteses and primary parathyroidism.

Management is with increased fluid intake, with diuretics (furosemide) once fluid volume is restored, treatment of the primary cause and specialist advice.

Magnesium
Magnesium is another mainly intracellular ion needed for energy storage and nerve transmission. It is closely associated with calcium and potassium function and produces similar symptoms – at low levels – of confusion, irritability, muscle weakness, arrhythmias and seizures.

Symptoms don't usually appear until levels are < 5.0 mmol/l.

Low magnesium levels can be due to excessive losses (e.g. gastrointestinal tract losses) or inadequate intake (e.g. starvation, alcoholism).

Intravenous supplementation (10–20 mmol $MgSO_4$) over 1–2 hours can be given. Magnesium supplementation to plasma levels of 1.5–2.0 mmol/l has also been used as a therapy for specific acute situations using the effects of increased magnesium levels to reduce seizures in pre-eclampsia, bronchospasm in asthma and to treat ventricular and supraventricular arrhythmias. Magnesium levels need close monitoring in this situation.

Renal function markers (acute) – urea and creatinine
The most immediate and important marker of renal function is urine output but this is also primarily affected by hypovolaemia and hypotension. An oliguric patient with rising creatinine and urea is likely to be in acute renal failure, which may initially be reversible but if allowed to continue will carry a high mortality risk and must be avoided if possible.

Common causes include hypovolaemia, infections, nephrotoxic drugs (e.g. non-steroidal anti-inflammatory drugs or Angiotensin converting enzyme inhibitors), rhabdomyolysis, and sepsis. Less common are vasculitic disease, glomerulonephritis, hepatorenal syndrome etc.

- *Urea* Urea is a product of breakdown of ammonia and depends upon adequate liver function for synthesis and renal function for excretion. Low levels of urea are associated with cirrhosis and high levels with renal failure.
  Normal levels of urea are 2.5–6.7 mmol/l – a high urea may indicate poor renal function when associated with high creatinine levels. On its own, a high urea level may indicate dehydration.

The ratio of urinary urea to plasma urea may help to differentiate the cause with a high ratio (10:1) when hypovolaemia causes the problem and a lower ratio (< 4:1) when the cause is renal.

- *Creatinine* Normal levels of creatinine are 70–110 µmol/l. These are affected by skeletal muscle mass, and low levels of creatinine are seen in starvation and the elderly. High levels occur in renal failure and rhabdomyolysis (muscle breakdown).

Acute renal impairment can commonly be resolved with adequate fluid replacement, treatment of the underlying cause (e.g. sepsis) and cessation of any nephrotoxic drugs.

Blood glucose

Levels can be monitored fairly accurately using bedside methods of measurement.

Management of blood glucose levels should be carried out according to local policy but usual levels to aim at are 4–8 mmol/l.

Infection and inflammation

The systemic inflammatory response (temperature, raised white cell count, increased heart rate and increased respiratory rate or carbon dioxide level) can be caused by infection, trauma, burns, pancreatitis, inhalation injury, massive blood loss, myocardial infarction, pulmonary embolus etc.

Box 8.1 gives the accepted definition of *systemic inflammatory response syndrome* (SIRS).

Box 8.1 Definition: SIRS

Two or more of the following:
- Temperature > 38 °C or < 36 °C
- Heart rate > 90 bpm
- Respiratory rate > 20 breaths/minute or $PaCO_2$ < 32 mmHg (4.3 kPa)
- White blood cells > 12×10^9/l, < 4×10^9/l or > 10% immature forms

---

When infection is the cause, this response is known as sepsis.

Other inflammatory markers are also used such as C-reactive protein (C-RP) or the number of neutrophils. A review of these markers will alert you to potential infection.

- **White blood cells (3.2–11.0×10^9/l):** The cell numbers are raised in acute infection or inflammation unless the infection is overwhelming or the patient is immunosuppressed, when they will be reduced.
- **Neutrophils (1.9–7.7×10^9/l)** are raised in bacterial infections, trauma, surgery, infarction, etc., but also in disseminated malignancy.
- **C-RP (0–10 mg/l)** is altered in a number of inflammatory conditions, with a response within hours of insult or infection and decrease in levels in 2–3 days of recovery.

Clear indicators of infection accompanied by your examination of the patient will allow some idea of likely sites of infection. A specimen for microscopy, culture and sensitivity will be required from all potential infection sites. You should check for the results of recent specimens sent to microbiology and if they have not been sent in the last 48 hours ensure that a specimen is collected and sent (Box 8.2).

Box 8.2 Common potential infection sites and microbiological specimens required

- Bacteraemia – blood cultures
- Chest – sputum sample
- Urinary tract – urine sample
- Wound/abscess – wound swab
- Drain – drain fluid

SUMMARY

Further assessment of the patient, once the priorities of airway, breathing and circulation have been assured, is essential. This will use both a further physical assessment of the whole patient and additional information from other sources such as the clinical record, the patient's charts and diagnostic investigations. This information allows a more comprehensive picture of what is happening to the patient to be built up. Visual information such as localised signs of inflammation or haemorrhage, palpation of areas of swelling or distension and reported patient history will all help to piece together what is happening. The patients charts include a lot of information, particularly if there is a trend of deterioration over several days. However, the accuracy of charts such as fluid balance have a major influence on the usefulness of the data. Electrolyte abnormalities, renal function indicators and inflammatory markers all help to build a bigger picture of the problem, and a working knowledge of the normal ranges of the indicators is important. Although initial assessment and response in the acute situation is focused on patient survival, unless the cause of the deterioration is identified it is unlikely that full recovery will occur.

CLINICAL SCENARIOS

Scenario 8.1

A 65-year-old man is admitted via A&E from a small care of the elderly hospital, where he has been treated for the past month for confusion. He has a past history of hypothyroid, poor renal function and bipolar affective disorder, for which he was taking lithium. His current lithium level is 1.7 (in the toxic range) and he has evidence of diabetes insipidus. His urea is 15.2 mmol/l, and his creatinine is 262 μmol/l. He is aggressive and confused, and records of his fluid intake and output are poor because of his behaviour. His respiratory rate is 20 breaths/minute; his SpO_2 is 95% on room air; his heart rate is 85 bpm; his blood pressure is 135/80 mmHg; and his temperature is 36.5 °C. His mouth is dry and his capillary refill time is 3 seconds.

Q1 What is your assessment and what problems are already evident for this gentleman?

Q2 What are potential problems for him?

Q3 *What would you suggest needs to be done at this stage?*

Overnight he is given temazepam and diazepam to help him to calm down and he becomes very drowsy.

Q4 *What would concern you about this treatment?*

By 07.00 the next morning he is unresponsive, with pinpoint pupils.

Q5 *What would you do?*

An intravenous infusion of 0.9% sodium chloride is commenced, and blood for full blood count, urea and electrolytes, and an arterial blood gas is taken.

Arterial blood gas (on air)

pH	7.327
pCO_2	5.6
pO_2	9.3
standard bicarbonate	21.2
Base excess	−3.4

Plasma sodium levels are 168 mmol/l. Plasma potassium is 3.5 mmol/l

Q6 *What would you do?*

Q7 *What are the possible causes of this high sodium level?*

Answers to scenario 8.1

Q1 • A – He does not appear to have an airway problem.
  • B – His respiratory observations are not abnormal at present; although respiratory rate is slightly high, this may be normal for him.
  • C – He appears to be fluid depleted with a slightly high heart rate, a prolonged CRT and a normal blood pressure. His fluid intake and output are unknown.
  • D – He is confused and his blood glucose should be checked
  • E – He has a degree of acute renal failure (urea is 15.2 mmol/l and creatinine is 262 μmol/L).

His problems are mild hypovolaemia and a degree of acute renal failure.

Q2 Further fluid volume depletion and further deterioration of renal function. He may also develop further deterioration in his conscious level.

Q3 Carbon dioxide levels are not known and it would be wise to undertake an ABG to establish these, as this is another potential cause of confusion. This will also inform you about the pH (potential acidosis and alkalosis) and the electrolytes.

If he is able to drink, then encourage increased oral fluids, start a fluid balance chart and maintain a strict record of fluid intake and output. If this is not possible due to behaviour, consider placing an intravenous cannula, and giving intravenous fluids and a urinary catheter to monitor urine output.

Review his drugs to identify any nephrotoxic agents.

Avoid further drugs, which may contribute to his confused state.

Take blood for a) full blood count, b)urea and electrolytes, c)liver function.

Q4 Benzodiazepines are excreted renally and will accumulate, causing respiratory depression, and possibly hypotension, which will contribute further to renal failure.

Q5 Immediate assessment and management of A–B–C–D–E. Airway protection if GCS < 8, give oxygen, correct hypotension with colloid, call for expert assistance (critical care outreach, senior member of the patient's medical team), suggest administering flumazenil (benzodiazepine antagonist), carry out further ABG.

Q6 As above and review the need for high-dependency care. His high sodium level should be treated with an infusion of 0.9% sodium chloride with the aim of reducing the sodium level slowly over 2–3days

Q7 The hypernatraemia could be due to his renal failure but may also be related to the high level of lithium (lithium toxicity), which will cause a nephrogenic diabetes insipidus causing him to lose water without salt and for sodium levels to rise. His confusion may also have caused further dehydration as a formal record of fluid balance was not possible.

Scenario 8.2

A 51-year-old lady is admitted from another local hospital for chemotherapy for recently diagnosed ovarian cancer. She has been on the previous ward for 5 days. She wakes in the middle of the night complaining of pain in her chest and some dyspnoea.

She is able to speak in short sentences.

Q1 *What would you do?*

Her respiratory rate is 35 breaths/minute and her SpO$_2$ is 93% on 50% oxygen via a humidified oxygen delivery system. Her breathing is laboured, with full use of accessory muscles. She coughs occasionally but does not produce any sputum. Air entry is equal on both sides of the chest and there are no added breath sounds. Her pulse is low in volume, rate 135 bpm and blood pressure is 95/60 mmHg. Her capillary refill time is 4 seconds and her peripheries (fingers) appear slightly blue and shut down.

She appears more comfortable with oxygen and the junior doctor who attends asks you to carry out a 12-lead ECG and prescribes intravenous opiate analgesia and some sub-lingual glyceryl trinitrate.

Q2 *What other possible causes could there be and what else would help to determine them?*

Q3 *What are the potential risks of the treatment prescribed by the junior doctor and what could you do to manage them?*

You decide to continue the full assessment of the patient and review the charts.She is talking to you and orientated to time and place. She tells you she has never had any heart problems before or experienced chest pain before.Her abdomen is slightly distended but not painful. As you examine the patient's legs, it becomes clear that her right calf is swollen and painful.

Q4 *What does this suggest?*

Answers to scenario 8.2

Q1 Carry out A, B, C of assessment (as above) and call for help. Commence oxygen via a non-rebreathe bag at B, sit patient upright if possible. Ensure IV access is functioning and get a bag of colloid ready.Continue on to D and E once help has arrived.

Q2 Other possible causes of sudden onset chest pain with shortness of breath are pulmonary embolus, pneumothorax, aortic dissection, and chest trauma.A chest x-ray is essential in determining other causes and should be ordered with the ECG. The patient's history is also an important part of understanding what is happening. A pulmonary embolus is associated with immobility, recent surgery, pelvic mass, malignant disease, oral contraceptive pill, childbirth, antiphospholipid syndrome, nephrotic syndrome.

Q3 The patient's blood pressure is low and it is possible that both the intravenous opiate and the glyceryl trinitrate would drop the blood pressure. Ensure that the intravenous fluid is running well and discuss this side effect of the treatment with the doctor prior to giving it. Monitor the blood pressure closely after the drug has been given and if necessary speed up the intravenous fluid to compensate.

Q4 The presence of unilateral painful calf-swelling in this situation is highly indicative of a deep vein thrombosis (DVT). The cause of the chest pain and shortness of breath is then likely to be a pulmonary embolus.

FURTHER READING

Adam S, Osborne S (2005) Critical Care Nursing: Science and Practice. Oxford University Press, p. 322

Ramrakha P, Moore K (2004) Oxford Handbook of Acute Medicine. Oxford University Press, pp. 570–583

Singer M, Webb AR (2005) Oxford Handbook of Critical Care. Oxford University Press, pp. 420–423

9 Patient-centred Care, Team Working and Communication

INTRODUCTION

In previous chapters we have seen how nurses can assess and manage acutely ill patients who deteriorate in hospital wards, using the A–B–C–D–E approach. This chapter will discuss issues that may arise after the initial treatment and rescue measures have been implemented. Firstly, tips will be given on how to call for more senior help, and the importance of a realistic management plan and effective documentation will be discussed. Team working and decision making will also be examined. Ongoing care when the decision to transfer a critically ill patient to a higher level of care will be discussed. Lastly, the patient in whom further interventions are deemed futile will be examined, including issues such as breaking bad news, end-of-life care and ethics.

LEARNING OBJECTIVES

By the end of this chapter you should be able to:

❑ Understand the importance of team working
❑ Understand the importance of verbal and written communication
❑ Discuss the decision-making process
❑ Effectively get help and describe a model for calling for assistance
❑ Understand basic ethical principles and describe a model for ethical decision making
❑ Discuss the important elements of safe patient transfer.

❏ Describe the important factors of breaking bad news and explain the care of patients at the end of their lives.

CALLING FOR HELP

Throughout this book, the importance of calling for more senior and expert help has been constantly emphasised, but the process of calling for help can be fraught with problems and misunderstanding. Each hospital or organisation will have its own calling procedures. These commonly involve the use of bleep systems, but the development of modern technology has meant an increase in the utilisation of Smart phones and ibleeps that incorporate the Internet and wireless technology. Some organisations will have rapid response teams, such as a Patient at Risk Team (PART) or Critical Care Outreach (CCO) teams, or use a hierarchy of clinical staff to respond to the deteriorating ward patient. It is important that the ward nurses are familiar with the phone or bleep systems and numbers in their own organisation. The cardiac arrest or 'crash call' telephone number was made 2222 throughout England and Wales in February 2004. The National Patient Safety Agency and the Resuscitation Council (UK) worked together to standardise the number to avoid confusion among staff who move between hospitals, and prevent delays in calling the cardiac arrest teams.

(www.npsa.nhs.uk/patientsafety/alerts-and-directives/alerts/crash-call/)

Key Point

The majority of hospitals in England and Wales now use the telephone number 2222 to alert the cardiac arrest team.

Some studies have reported that nurses can feel anxious about calling a doctor when they are concerned about a patient, in case they say the wrong thing; they fear looking stupid or being ridiculed (Cioffi 2000; Andrews and Waterman 2005). The language used by nurses and doctors can be fundamentally different and when talking about acutely unwell patients misunderstandings and confusion can occur. Nurses tend to use social language, which is descriptive and subjective, while doctors use medical terms that tend to include objective terms. A nurse might say that the 'patient feels unwell and looks pale', while the doctor might to refer to this patient as being 'peripherally shut down, with a capillary refill time of greater than 3 seconds'. This difference in language use may cause ineffective communication, resulting in doctors not grasping the urgency of the situation, and nursing staff feeling frustrated. Early warning scoring systems (discussed in Chapter 2) may help with communication, providing a universal language that can be used by all grades of staff, but it is important that clinical staff are able to get messages across in a succinct and effective manner. Some tips for calling for help are outlined in Box 9.1.

Box 9.1 Tips for calling for help

- Before bleeping a doctor, make sure you have all the information you need to hand.
- When bleeping a doctor, stay by the phone to receive the call back.
- State your name, position, and where you are located.
- State the patient's name, age and diagnosis.
- State the current problem, giving observation and assessment findings (Use SBAR – see Box 9.2.)
- Be clear about what you are expecting the doctor to do.
- Do not hesitate to call the cardiac arrest team if the patient has collapsed, or if the patient is rapidly deteriorating or you have any major concerns.

The Institute for Innovation and Improvement (www.institute.nhs.uk/) gives information about the Situation, Background, Assessment and Recommendation (SBAR) model for communication that has been widely adopted in the UK. The SBAR model is a technique that provides a framework for communication between members of the healthcare team (Box 9.2).

Box 9.2 The SBAR communication model (www.
institute.nhs.uk/)

Situation
- Identify yourself and the site/unit you are calling from
- Identify the patient by name and the reason for your report
- Describe your concern

Background
- Give the patient's reason for admission
- Explain any significant medical history
- Inform the physician of the patient's background: admitting
  diagnosis, date of admission, prior procedures, current medications, allergies, pertinent laboratory results and other relevant diagnostic results

Assessment
- Current vital signs
- Clinical impressions and concerns

Recommendation
- Explain what you need – be specific about request and time
  frame
- Make suggestions
- Clarify expectations

Reproduced under the terms of the Click-Use Licence

The steps of SBAR make it clear that any healthcare worker
calling for help needs to have certain vital information immediately to hand before making the call. Taking the time to collect
this information and assessing the situation may seem to be
taking extra time, in what is a stressful, critical situation. However,
having the extra information may make a difference in the quality
of information given to the doctor and being able to convince
them of the critical state of the patient. The doctor may also be
able to make suggestions about immediate treatment measures,
such as increasing fluids or turning up inspired oxygen levels.
These can be instigated by the nurse while waiting for the arrival
of the medical team. Effective communication means that doctors

have the information they need to prioritise which patients they need to see, what treatments or interventions they may need to commence when they get to the patient, or whether they may need to call for more expert help themselves.

Unless the patient is so unwell that you feel you have to physically stay with them, it is best not to delegate the call for help to someone else unless you are sure that person has all the relevant information, and the confidence to ensure the message is received and understood. It is not unusual to receive calls for help from nurses who do not know the patient's name, or the last set of vital signs, and are unclear about what it is they want done for the patient. These muddled communication practices can lead to frustration and misunderstanding between the healthcare team and could result in a delay in effective treatment for the patient.

Key Point

Remember – if you are concerned that a patient is rapidly deteriorating, or you have doubts about your competency to cope with the situation, don't hesitate to put out a cardiac arrest call.

TEAM WORKING

The smooth running of the hospital organisation and the delivery of clinical care are improved when effective team working is evident (Jackson, 1998). The efficient assessment and initial management of a deteriorating patient may necessitate the input of a range of clinical expertise. The traditional model of medical care in UK hospitals has been for the patient to be cared for under a specific medical consultant and his team. Medical teams are becoming increasingly specialised and the legislation around Working Time Directives (www.healthcareworkforce.nhs.uk/ workingtimedirective.html) has seen doctors' weekly hours reduced to 58, with a further reduction to 48 hours in 2009. This has resulted in a change in doctors' working patterns. Doctors are now more likely to work in shift patterns, and the need for effective team working among the wider multidisciplinary team is paramount to ensure effective communication and streamlined care between specialists as well as between shifts. The patient will benefit from the expertise of other healthcare workers in the multidisciplinary team. From critical care doctors to palliative care nursing, teams can work well together if there is mutual professional respect and the patient's needs are put at the centre of care.

Junior and inexperienced healthcare staff caring for acutely ill patients who are deteriorating need appropriate support and expert advice. However, there is evidence that there can be a delay in consultants and other experts getting involved in the care of deteriorating patients. The National Confidential Enquiry into Patient Outcome and Death (NCEPOD, 2005) reported in a study of medical patients who were admitted to the intensive care unit (ICU) that junior doctors failed to seek further advice in 30% of the 560 patients who went on to die in ICU. Consultant physicians had no knowledge or input into the referrals of 57% of 1130 cases that were transferred to ICU. The reasons for the failures in the system are numerous and complex. McQuillan et al (1998) reported in a study of 100 emergency admissions of ward patients to ICU that 54% received suboptimal ward care due to failure of the organisation, lack of knowledge, failure to appreciate clinical urgency, lack of supervision and failure to seek advice.

Effective team work is key to the success of organisational change, and involves shared goals, mutual trust and respect, and the sharing of ideas in an open atmosphere (NHS Modernisation Agency, 2003). Effective decision making is dependent on shared knowledge and clinical experience. Deteriorating ward patients need the involvement of healthcare staff with those qualities in order that they make meaningful decisions about their care.

DECISION MAKING AND PLANNING CARE

Clinical decision making is an extremely complex process and can be further compounded in the stressful situation of a deteriorating acutely unwell patient. The process of making decisions about patient care is similar to making decisions about any other aspects of life.

We need to:

- **assess** the situation so that we can
- **diagnose** what the problem is; then we need to
- **plan** how we are deal with the situation, which we then
- **implement**, followed by a period when we
- **evaluate**.

The process can be cyclical and dynamic, especially in healthcare where new information may be presenting itself all the time and the patient's response to treatment can be unpredictable.

At each stage of the decision making process the clinician needs to consider a number of factors:

- What is in the patient's best interests?
- Are you the best person to be making the decision?
- What is known about the situation? What facts do you have? What information might be missing?
- What is your 'gut' feeling or intuition about the situation?
- What are risks?
- What are the benefits?
- Are there any unconventional solutions you could consider?

Considering the process of decision making, it follows that healthcare staff with more experience and greater knowledge will make better decisions. Experience involves the repeated exposure of the individual to similar situations over months or years, where pattern recognition is developed and intuitive reasoning becomes a feature of the experienced nurse or doctor. This may be problematical in the recognition of the critically ill ward patient, where nurses and doctors may have expert knowledge and experience in their specialist areas, but have had minimal and infrequent exposure to critically ill patients. Critical healthcare decisions are complex and usually made in highly stressful situations, characterised by constant interruptions, distractions and competing resources. A systematic approach to assessment, diagnosis, planning, implementation and evaluation, coupled with a team approach involving good communication and record keeping, will all help improve the quality of decision making and enhance communication.

Making decisions about patient care needs to involve the patients themselves as well as their families and loved ones. This can be difficult when the patient is acutely unwell and deteriorating, or is so critically ill that they may not be able to communicate effectively or understand what is being said to them. Every effort must be made to consider the patient's wishes at each stage of the decision-making process, and communicate care decisions to the patient and their families in the most appropriate way.

ASSESSING MENTAL CAPACITY

Recent legislation in the Mental Capacity Act (www.opsi.gov. uk/ACTS/acts2005/ukpga_20050009_en_1) has outlined and updated the legal framework that addresses capacity and decision making when dealing with health, social care and finances. The Act aims to provide protection for individuals and staff, powers to make decisions and take action and outline the duties of staff and carers. The Act came into force in April 2007 and contains five underlying principles – see Box 9.3.

Box 9.3 Five principles of the Mental Capacity Act

1. A person must be assumed to have capacity unless it is established that they lack capacity.
2. A person is not to be treated as unable to make a decision unless all practicable steps to help him to do so have been taken without success.
3. A person is not to be treated as unable to make a decision merely because he takes an unwise decision.
4. An act done, or a decision made, under this Act for or on behalf of a person who lacks capacity must be done, or made, in his best interests.
5. Before the act is done, or the decision is made, regard must be had to whether the purpose for which it is needed can be as effectively achieved in a way that is less restrictive of the person's rights and freedom of action.

There are clear guidelines in the Act regarding the test for mental capacity (see Box 9.4) and clinicians are expected to adhere to this test and clearly document the process and outcome in the patient's notes.

Box 9.4 Guidelines to assess mental capacity

A person must be able to:
1. Understand the information relevant to the decision.
   - The nature, purposes and consequences of their decision.
   - Understand information in broad terms and simple language.
   - Can consult others for help.
2. Retain the information.
   - Able to retain the information long enough to make the decision.
   - Can use aids to help retain information such as recordings, books and notes.
3. Use or weigh the information as part of the decision-making process.
   - Believe the information
4. Communicate the decision.
   - Communicate in any understandable way such as hand squeezing or blinking.
   - Can be assisted in communication steps.

The assessment of a person's capacity is time specific in that it relates to a specific time and may change over time. Capacity also relates to a specific decision and may vary depending on the decision. Capacity should not be solely based on appearance, age, behaviour or condition.

In emergency medical situations, urgent decisions need to be made without delay, and the principle of acting in the person's best interest will apply. Clinicians must still attempt to communicate with the patient to ensure they are doing all they can to inform the patient about what decisions are being made about their care. Where possible information should be sought from the patient's friends and family to find out what the patient's beliefs and values might be in the current situation. However, doctors are under no obligation to provide life-sustaining treatment if they believe it is not in the best interests of the patient, even if it will result in the patient's death. In a dispute regarding these decisions, the Court of protection may need to be consulted.

Further information about the Mental Capacity Act can be found at www.dca.gov.uk/legal-policy/mental-capacity.

ETHICS

Ethical issues and dilemmas will always be at the centre of clinical decision making in healthcare. The inherent principles that underpin healthcare are those of:

- respect for persons
- beneficence (doing good)
- non-maleficence (doing no harm)
- veracity (truth telling)
- justice.

Healthcare staff are constantly striving to uphold these principles while adhering to demands for efficiency in a climate of resource limitation. Clinical decision making can be complicated by the different values and belief systems of all the people involved, limited resources available and the demands of other patients in the system. By their very nature, these decisions can evoke powerful emotions and cause considerable stress to all involved. An ethical decision-making model developed by Uustal (1990) is presented here in Box 9.5 as an aid to reduce the stress and bias inherent in the decision-making process.

Box 9.5 Clinical Ethical Decision Making Model (Uustal, 1990)

1. Identify the problem.
- Who are the people involved?
- How are they interrelated?
- What is involved?
- Identify the values/ethical dilemmas.

Make a concise statement of the problem, stating the

Box 9.5 (cont'd)

conflicts.

2. **State your values and ethical position. Explore the patient's values.**
   - The patient's choices should be the primary focus of the direction of decision making. The nurse should communicate these choices to others in the healthcare team.
   - If your own values conflict with those of the patient, it may be that you should replace yourself as the patient's primary care-giver.
   - Identify the ethical principles that are inherently important in the dilemma, and rank order. This will help identify the primary ethical principle that will influence your decisions and behaviour.

3. **Generate alternatives for resolving the dilemma.**
   Use a brainstorming technique. Do not pass judgement on any alternatives at this stage. If possible, involve the patient and relatives and all health carers involved.

4. **Examine and categorise the alternatives.**
   Examine those that are consistent and those that are inconsistent with your values, and those of the patient.

5. **Predict the possible consequences of those acceptable alternatives.**
   For each alternative, predict its physical, psychological, social, spiritual and short- and long-term consequences according to the patient's standpoint.

6. **Prioritise the acceptable alternatives.**
   Which have the most merit in the given situation? Rank order the alternatives. If it is difficult, choose the alternative that breaks the fewest ethical principles, or results in the least harm, or greatest good for the patient.

7. **Develop a plan of action.**

8. **Implement the plan**
   Communicate with all involved.

9. **Evaluate the action taken**
   Ask yourself: 'Did I do the right thing?' 'Were my actions ethical?' All should be involved in the evaluation.
   Would you repeat your actions if you came across the same situation again? If 'yes', then good. If 'no', then recheck steps 1 and 3, and continue through the stages.

This article was published in *Critical Care Nursing Clinics of North America* 2(3), Uustal, Diann B., 'Enhancing your ethical reasoning', pp. 437–442. Copyright Elsevier 1990.

DOCUMENTATION

The process of care and decision making should be underpinned by clear, structured documentation in the patient's hospital notes at every stage. The NCEPOD report (2005) found that medical notes were poorly written and consequently made a number of recommendations for improving the quality of record keeping:

- All entries in the notes should be dated and timed and should be signed, and end with a legible name, status and contact number (bleep or telephone).
- Each entry should clearly identify the name and grade of the most senior doctor involved in the patient episode.
- Resuscitation status should be documented in patients who are at risk of deterioration.
- Each trust should audit compliance with this recommendation by regular review of patients who suffered a cardiac arrest and assessment of whether a 'do not attempt resuscitation' order should have been made prior to this event.

(NCEPOD, 2005, p. 4)

Recent recommendations from the National Institute for Health and Clinical Excellence (NICE, 2007) also underline the importance of a clear written monitoring plan and a formal structured handover of care. Documentation can be further complicated by professionals holding specific notes about the patient in different locations. Nursing and other allied health profession's documentation located separately from the main medical notations can contribute to confusion and missed information for the doctor. The patient's notes should be a consecutive record of all care and decision making by all the multidisciplinary team.

Key Point

The quality of your documentation reflects your expertise and professionalism. Make sure your records are legible, dated, timed and signed.

HANDOVER

The shift handover process has long been the domain of the nurse, but the changing working patterns of doctors with the European Working Time Directives have necessitated a move to shift working for medical teams.

One communication process model suggested by Weinfeld and Donohue (1989) suggests that communication contains six basic steps, and these can be interpreted through the handover of a patient's care:

1. The (sender) healthcare worker formulates an idea about the patient's care based on their experiences during the shift.
2. The ideas are encoded by the healthcare worker and put into some sort of symbolic form; language or written.
3. The message is transmitted through the handover process by speech or by the written notes.
4. The (receiver) healthcare worker perceives the message.
5. The receiver healthcare worker decodes the message and translates the meaning to fit into their frame of reference.
6. The receiver feeds back to the sender that the message has been received and understood.

Throughout this process we can see that the practice of communication is complex and has the potential for misunderstanding and individual interpretation at each of the six steps. The handover of patient care from one set of healthcare staff to another has the potential to threaten patient safety issues; important patient communication may be misinterpreted or simply not take place. However, the handover is also a learning opportunity where nurses and doctors can exchange their knowledge, support each other, and systematic errors may be detected by a 'fresh pair of eyes'.

The handover process is not only a communication tool for patient care issues, but also an important signal that marks the beginning or an end to a shift where teams can hand over, or take on, the responsibility of patient care. Teams working together establish their roles and assign duties, or debrief and reflect on the shift just worked, highlighting areas of good practice and discussing where improvements can be made. Operational issues can also be discussed at these times, and solutions can be agreed to actual and potential problems that may arise during the coming shift. Having a specific structure, a dedicated space and protected time to hand over patient care will all enhance the quality of the communication process.

TRANSFERRING THE PATIENT

Once the deteriorating patient has been appropriately assessed and initial treatment measures have been implemented, the decision may be made that it is necessary to move them to an area that is better equipped to care for them, depending on their medical problem. A patient who has suffered a cardiac arrest and requires ventilation will need to go to a level three area. A patient who has had a myocardial infarction may need to be transferred to a cardiac care unit. A patient may also need to be transferred to undergo a specific procedure or investigation, such as an operation or x-ray. It may also be necessary to transfer the patient to another hospital if the current hospital does not possess the required specialist expertise that the patient may need, such as neurological care or cardiac surgery.

The transfer of an acutely ill patient poses some considerable risks that could result in death of the patient. A study of 191 Australian incident reports (Beckmann et al, 2004) related to intra-hospital transport found 900 contributing factors to critical incidents during transfer, 46% system based and 54% human based, including:

- Communication problems
- Inadequate protocols
- Inadequate training
- Equipment problems
- Failure to recognise problems
- Inadequate preparation of the patient
- Haste and inattention.

In the UK, the Intensive Care Society (ICS, 2002) have developed transfer guidelines that apply to the transfer of critically ill patients both within and between hospitals. The prime aim of the transfer process is the patient's safety.

All aspects of the patient's transfer need to be considered and planned by healthcare personnel with the right experience and skill, and who are able to make decisions about treatment and where the patient is to be cared for. The first consideration is whether the patient should be transferred at all, and each decision should be weighed up considering the risks and benefits to the patient.

Special care should be taken to ensure the patient is adequately stabilised prior to the transfer; that they have the right equipment and supplies for their journey, taking into account any complications that may occur; and that the right healthcare staff with appropriate skills accompany the patient. A checklist for transfer can be seen in Table 9.1. Records should be completed, and any information needed for a smooth handover should be included in the notes. A plan of care should be included that documents appropriate resuscitation decisions. All documentation should be collected together to accompany the patient, as well as the patient's personal belongings. The patient and his family should be involved in the decision to transfer, and be kept fully informed about the transfer process, including any information they might need about where the patient is going to be cared for.

Key Point

Before you leave on a transfer make sure you are happy that the patient is stable, you have the right equipment and the accompanying personnel have the right experience and competence.

BREAKING BAD NEWS

Having to impart bad news to a patient or their family is an inevitable part of care when dealing with acutely unwell and deteriorating patients. How this is done has a lasting impact on the recipients of the news, and will have a profound effect on how they accept and deal with the situation. Difficult conversations should be carefully considered and adequately prepared. Care should be taken that all the information required is available to the doctor who will be talking to the patient or their relatives.

Table 9.1 Checklist for patient transfer.
Reproduced from Intensive Care Society (2002) *Guidelines for the transport of the critically ill adult*, with permission.

Is the patient stable for transport?		Are you ready for departure?	
Airway	✓	*Patient*	✓
Airway safe or secured by intubation		Stable on transport trolley	
Tracheal tube position confirmed on chest x-ray		Appropriately monitored	
Ventilation	✓	All infusions running and lines adequately secured	
Paralysed, sedated and ventilated		Adequately sedated and paralysed	
Ventilation established on transport ventilator		Adequately secured to trolley	
Adequate gas exchange confirmed by arterial blood gas		Adequately wrapped to prevent heat loss	
Circulation	✓	**Staff**	✓
Heart rate, BP stable		Adequately trained and experienced	
Tissue and organ perfusion adequate		Received appropriate handover	
Any obvious blood loss controlled		Adequately clothed and insured	
Circulating blood volume restored		**Equipment**	✓
Haemoglobin adequate		Appropriately equipped ambulance	
Minimum of two routes of venous access		Appropriate equipment and drugs	
Arterial line and central venous access if appropriate		Batteries checked (spare batteries available)	
Neurology	✓	Sufficient oxygen supplies	
Seizures controlled, metabolic causes excluded		Portable phone charged and available	
Raised intracranial pressure appropriately managed		Money/credit cards for emergencies	
Trauma	✓	**Organisation**	✓
Cervical spine protected		Case notes, x-rays, results, blood collected	
Pneumothoraces drained		Transfer documentation prepared	
Intrathoracic and intra-abdominal bleeding controlled		Location of bed and receiving doctor known	

Table 9.1 (cont'd)

Is the patient stable for transport?		Are you ready for departure?	
Intra-abdominal injuries adequately investigated and appropriately managed		Receiving unit advised of departure time and estimated time of arrival	
Long bone/pelvic fractures stabilised		Telephone numbers of referring and receiving units available	
Metabolic	✓	Relatives informed	
Blood glucose > 4 mmol/l		Return travel arrangements in place	
Potassium < 6 mmol/l		Ambulance crew briefed	
Ionised calcium > 1 mmol/l		Police escort arranged if appropriate	
Acid–base balance acceptable		**Departure**	✓
Temperature maintained		Patient trolley secured	
Monitoring	✓	Electrical equipment plugged into ambulance power supply	
ECG		Ventilator transferred to ambulance oxygen supply	
Blood pressure		All equipment safely mounted or stowed	
Oxygen saturation		Staff seated and wearing seat belts	
End tidal carbon dioxide			
Temperature			

Source: Intensive Care Society (2002), Appendices 3 and 4

As with the communication process outlined above, communicating bad news to anxious patients and their families will have inherent risks that may result in misunderstanding, additional stress and unrealistic expectations. Care needs be taken that the person receiving the news has had their cultural and religious differences taken into consideration and that the language used has been adapted to the age and intellect of the recipient if necessary.

Smith (2003) recommends the following guidance when having to break bad news.

- Ensure the correct environment (e.g. a private comfortable room).
- Tissues, drinks, a telephone and relevant written information should be to hand.

- Allow time so that the interview is unhurried.
- Avoid interruptions by leaving bleeps and pagers with someone outside who can answer them.
- Ensure all relevant information is to hand. Be familiar with patient's past and current history.
- Introduce yourself and explain your role.
- Ensure you know each family member and their relation to the patient.
- Establish what is already known and understood about the situation by the patient and their family.
- Be honest.
- Avoid euphemisms and jargon.
- Try to use a 'warning shot' (e.g. 'I'm afraid I have some bad news').
- Be aware of body language.
- Allow time for patients and relatives to think, reflect and ask questions.
- Check the patient's and their family's understanding of the information and reassure them that you can meet again to discuss the situation.

It is important that conversations with patients and their families are recorded in the patients medical notes so that other clinicians can be kept informed of the situation and subsequent discussions with the patient and family can be consistent.

END-OF-LIFE CARE

It is inevitable that some patients who deteriorate on the ward will not recover in spite of the resuscitative measures and efforts of the critical care team. There are strong recommendations by NCEPOD (2005) that treatment limitation decisions and 'do not attempt resuscitation' (DNAR) orders should be considered in patients who are at the terminal stages of an illness, where the disease processes are unlikely to be reversed, or where the patient's pre-morbid state does not give them sufficient physiological reserve to survive any further deterioration. These sorts of decisions are difficult to discuss with patients and their families, but they should be discussed in a timely manner when the patient may still have sufficient mental capacity to enable them to participate in the decision-making process. Waiting until the patient is critically unwell is often too late and treatment decisions at that time may not be in the best interests of the patient. Many patients are resuscitated, involving aggressive and invasive measures such as cardiac massage and tracheal intubation, only to have a DNAR decision made immediately after the event. Many patients who have life-limiting chronic disease may have already had discussions with their families about end-of-life care, and many patients are aware when the end of their life is near. Having the opportunity to have open and frank discussions about the situation can give the patient back a sense of control, and reassurance that fears such as pain and discomfort can be managed.

Treatment decisions need not necessarily be an 'all or nothing' choice. Over 30 years ago, a group of physicians classified four categories of intervention based on the patient's prognosis:

1. Maximum therapy without reservation
2. Maximum therapy with daily evaluation
3. Selective limitation of life-saving therapies
4. All therapy discontinued.

(Clinical Care Committee of Massachusetts
General Hospital, 1976)

There still seems to be a reluctance to make treatment limitation decisions for patients on the general wards for fear that the patient may not receive any interventions or access to critical care expertise. Treatment limitation decisions are closely associated with 'Do not attempt resuscitation' (DNAR) decisions, with resulting confusion and misunderstanding regarding the aims of care. DNAR decisions refer to actions to be taken in the case of a patient suffering a cardiorespiratory arrest (CRA). CRA is defined as cessation of breathing and an absence of a pulse, and patients who suffer an unexpected in-hospital cardiac arrest where resuscitation is attempted have a very poor outcome. In a study of over 14,000 inpatients who had a CRA, Peberdy et al (2003) reported that although 44% patients had a return of spontaneous circulation after the arrest, only 17% survived to hospital discharge. Many inpatients who survive CRA are left significantly compromised, requiring considerable ongoing treatment and care. DNAR decisions made with patients and their families can offer realistic plans of care, and should not automatically deny the patient other life-saving or symptom relieving interventions. Some patients with DNAR decisions can benefit from non-invasive ventilation and admission to intensive care, but care plans need to be made with multidisciplinary team involvement. The patient should have explicit treatment plans documented in the medical notes with decision rationales and alternative solutions recorded in the event of a change in the patient's condition. DNAR and treatment limitation decisions should be regularly reviewed and updated.

The British Medical Association with the Resuscitation Council and Royal College of Nursing published guidance in 2007 on resuscitation decisions (www.resus.org.uk/pages/dnar.htm) and highlighted the main considerations when making these difficult decisions, which have been outlined in Box 9.6.

Box 9.6 Main messages regarding decisions about cardiopulmonary resuscitation (CPR). Reproduced from Decisions Relating to Cardiopulmonary Resuscitation, BMA, 2007, with permission.

- Decisions about CPR must be made on the basis of an individual assessment of each patient's case.
- Advance care planning, including making decisions about CPR, is an important part of good clinical care for those at risk of cardiorespiratory arrest.
- Communication and the provision of information are essential parts of good quality care.
- It is not necessary to initiate discussion about CPR with a patient if there is no reason to believe that the patient is likely to suffer a cardiorespiratory arrest.
- Where no explicit decision has been made in advance there should be an initial presumption in favour of CPR.
- If CPR would not re-start the heart and breathing, it should not be attempted.
- Where the expected benefit of attempted CPR may be outweighed by the burdens, the patient's informed views are of paramount importance. If the patient lacks capacity, those

---

Box 9.6 (cont'd)

close to the patient should be involved in discussions to explore the patient's wishes, feelings, beliefs and values.

- If a patient with capacity refuses CPR, or a patient lacking capacity has a valid and applicable advance decision refusing CPR, this should be respected.
- A Do Not Attempt Resuscitation (DNAR) decision does not override clinical judgement in the unlikely event of a reversible cause of the patient's respiratory or cardiac arrest that does not match the circumstances envisaged.
- DNAR decisions apply only to CPR and not to other aspects of treatment.

www.resus.org.uk/pages/dnar.htm

CARE OF THE DYING PATIENT

When the decision has been made to discontinue aggressive therapy and implement end-of-life caring measures, the clinical team can use the guidance contained in the Liverpool Care Pathway (LCP) (www.mcpcil.org.uk/liverpoolcarepathway). The LCP was developed at the Royal Liverpool University Hospital with the Marie Curie Centre and has been recommended for widespread implementation by the Department of Health.

The aim of the LCP programme is to improve the quality of care at the end of life for all patients and enable more patients to live and die in the place of their choice (www.endoflifecare.nhs.uk/eolc). There are three main components to the LCP in the care of the dying patient:

1. *Initial assessment and care goals*
   - *Comfort measures*
   - *Psychological insight*
   - *Religious/Spiritual support*
   - *Communication*
   - *Summary*
2. *Ongoing care goals*
   - *Comfort measures*
   - *Treatment /procedures*
   - *Medication*
   - *Mobility/pressure area care*

- *Bowel care*
- *Psychological/Insight support*
- *Religious/spiritual support*
3. *Care after death goals*
   - *Communication with GP*
   - *Laying out procedures*
   - *Family/others information*
   - *Property and belongings*
   - *Bereavement information*

(Ellershaw and Wilkinson, 2003)

The patient and their family, with the primary medical team, the critical care team, and the palliative care team, can all work together to ensure appropriate decisions are made and recorded so as to ensure that the best possible care for the patient is achieved.

CHAPTER SUMMARY

This chapter has explored areas of care that may arise following the assessment and initial management of the deteriorating acutely ill ward patient. Following an acute episode of care, the decision may be taken to transfer the patient to a higher level of care, continue to actively treat the patient on the ward, or to change the aim of care to comfort measures in preparation for the end of life. Team working is at the heart of quality patient care and issues such as communication, decision making and documentation are key to effective care practices.

REFERENCES

Andrews T, Waterman H (2005) Packaging: A grounded theory of how to report physiological deterioration effectively. Journal of Advanced Nursing 52(5):473–481

Beckmann U, Gillies DM, et al (2004) Incidents relating to the intra-hospital transfer of critically ill patients. An analysis of the reports submitted to the Australian Incident Monitoring Study in Intensive Care. Intensive Care Medicine 30(8):1579–1585

Cioffi J (2000) Nurses' experiences of making decisions to call emergency assistance to their patients. Journal of Advanced Nursing 32(1):108–114

Clinical Care Committee of Massachusetts General Hospital (1976) The New England Journal of Medicine 295(7):362–364

Ellershaw J, Wilkinson S (2003) Care of the Dying. Oxford University Press. Oxford

ICS (2002) Guidelines for the transport of the critically ill adult. Intensive Care Society, London

Jackson S (1998) Organisational effectiveness within National Health Service (NHS) Trusts. International Journal of Health Care Quality Assurance Incorporating Leadership Health Services 11(6–7):216–221

McQuillan P, Pilkington S, et al (1998) Confidential inquiry into quality of care before admission to intensive care. British Medical Journal 316(7148):1853–1858

NCEPOD (2005) An Acute Problem? National Confidential Enquiry into Patient Outcome and Death, London

NICE (2007) Acutely Ill Patients in Hospital. National Institute for Health and Clinical Excellence, London

NHS Modernisation Agency (2003) Teamworking for improvement: Planning for spread and sustainability. Report No. 5. Modernisation Agency, London

Peberdy MA, Kaye W, et al (2003) Cardiopulmonary resuscitation of adults in the hospital: A report of 14720 cardiac arrests from the National Registry of Cardiopulmonary Resuscitation. Resuscitation 58(3):297–308

Smith G (2003) ALERT. Acute Life-Threatening Events Recognition and Treatment. University of Portsmouth.

Uustal DB (1990) Enhancing Your Ethical Reasoning. Critical Care Nursing Clinics of North America 2(3):437–442

Weinfeld RS, Donohue EM (1989) Communicating Like a Manager. Williams and Wilkins, Baltimore.

Appendix 1: Acid–Base Balance and Arterial Blood Gases

The human body usually works to keep its internal contents and functions operating within quite narrow limits – for instance, temperature, blood pressure and the different quantities of fluids and electrolytes in the body are normally very tightly regulated. Maintenance of the balance between acid and base in the body is another key mechanism; and acute illness is frequently associated with changes in this balance.

Our understanding of the means by which acid and base are generated and interact is incomplete, and there are several sometimes conflicting theories about exactly how this happens. However, analysis of acid, base and related measures such as arterial blood gases can often help clarify the nature of an acute illness and also the severity of that illness. This section describes how acid is generated and processed in the body, some common disorders, and a standard approach to help determine what is happening in particular patients with abnormal acid–base balance.

PRODUCTION OF ACID IN THE BODY

Waste products from everyday body metabolism continually generate acid – for example, by the breakdown of foodstuffs into substances such as carbon dioxide (CO_2). CO_2 is not in itself an acid, but 20,000 mmol of CO_2 may be produced daily and some of this constant stream of CO_2 combines with water ($CO_2 + H_2O$) to create carbonic acid (H_2CO_3). Carbonic acid is actually a relatively weak acid, but is significant because there can be so much of it in the body.

Acids are chemical compounds containing active hydrogen ions (that is, the H^+ part of H_2CO_3). Fluids with high concentrations of hydrogen ions are strong acids. The hydrogen ion content of fluids – including blood – can be measured using the pH scale, which ranges from 0 to 14. Fluids with the highest concentrations of hydrogen ions have low pH values. Those with low concentrations of hydrogen ions have high pH values: these are alkali. The terms base and alkali are used more or less interchangeably, although strictly speaking alkalis are base substances dissolved in water. As the human body is mostly composed of water, base in the body will generally be alkali.

Different body fluids have different pH values. For example, gastric acid may have a pH as low as 1 or 2 (i.e. it is a strong acid), while urinary pH typically ranges from 4.6 (medium strength acid) to 8.0 (a weak alkali). The pH of blood is normally between 7.35 and 7.45: if the measured pH of a blood sample is lower than 7.35 the patient is said to be acidaemic; while if the pH is higher than 7.45, the patient is alkalaemic. Acidaemia and alkalaemia are signs of significant disease, and are also harmful in themselves as normal enzyme activity and cellular function are adversely affected by altered pH. Acidemia can result in central nervous system (CNS) and cardiovascular depression, while alkalaemia is associated with CNS hypersensitivity, seizures and also, eventually, reduced consciousness.

CONTROL OF ACID LEVELS

The body uses several mechanisms to eliminate or neutralise acid. Most of the CO_2 produced by cellular metabolism is normally eliminated during expiration: these quantities of CO_2 are not then available to create excessive carbonic acid. Because CO_2 is continually produced, effective respiratory function is absolutely crucial to acid–base balance. Acute or chronic lung disease puts the patient at risk from inadequate clearance of CO_2 (i.e. CO_2 retention and respiratory acidosis).

The body also eliminates acid in urine; as seen above, the pH of urine is generally lower than that of blood, indicating that the kidneys tend to selectively remove hydrogen ions from the blood. But, if there is renal failure, as frequently happens in severe acute illness, fewer hydrogen ions may be eliminated by the kidneys, bringing about a renal acidosis.

Some acid in the body is not eliminated, but is made less potent by being 'buffered' in chemical combinations that reduce hydrogen ion activity. For example, excess free hydrogen ions in the blood (H^+) may be combined with bicarbonate (HCO_3^-) to create the relatively weak carbonic acid.[1]

The body retains a store of buffers like bicarbonate to help control acid levels, so if these stores become depleted, free acid will tend to accumulate and acidaemia may result. There are normally 22–26 mmol/l of bicarbonate in arterial blood. Lower levels of bicarbonate indicate that either bicarbonate is being lost from the body (e.g. due to profuse diarrhoea or other gastrointestinal losses); or that the bicarbonate is being consumed in buffering an increased production of acid.

Importantly, the body is able to increase its bicarbonate levels in disease states where there are chronically high levels of acid production. This is the case in COPD patients who typically have elevated CO_2 values and therefore a tendency to generate more acid than people without COPD. Over time, these patients also increase the bicarbonate content of their blood, so that the raised CO_2 is compensated by raised bicarbonate and the blood pH is kept in the normal range.

RESPIRATORY CAUSES OF ACID–BASE IMBALANCE

It is to be expected that there is always *some* CO_2 in the blood. The normal range of CO_2 in arterial blood (pCO_2) is 4.6–6.1 kPa. A pCO_2 greater than 6.1 kPa (e.g. in Type 2 respiratory failure) causes *respiratory acidosis*. Everything else being equal, pH will be

---

[1] It can be seen that there is a complex relationship between carbon dioxide (CO_2), water (H_2O), carbonic acid (H_2CO_3), bicarbonate (HCO_3^-), and hydrogen ions (H^+). Carbonic acid – an acid, provides the ingredients for the creation of bicarbonate – a base. These are components of the carbonic acid/bicarbonate buffer system in which different chemical combinations are created to take up or free hydrogen ions to maintain pH within a narrow normal range depending on conditions in the body at a particular point. This relationship is sometimes written as $CO_2 + H_2O \rightleftharpoons H_2CO_3 \rightleftharpoons HCO_3^- + H^+$ (the $\rightleftharpoons$ symbol indicating that buffering processes can move from left to right beginning with carbon dioxide combining with water, or from right to left with hydrogen ions joining with bicarbonate).

reduced. At the most basic level, treatment of acute respiratory acidosis is aimed at helping the patient to breathe more deeply and/or more quickly, and at ensuring that gaseous exchange is not compromised by reduced lung volumes, excessive secretions or fluid.

A pCO_2 less than 4.6 kPa (e.g. in a patient that is hyperventilating) causes *respiratory alkalosis*. Everything else being equal, because there is less CO_2 – and less acid – than usual in the blood, the pH will tend to rise.

METABOLIC CAUSES OF ACID–BASE IMBALANCE

Changes in acid–base balance not due to abnormal CO_2 levels are caused by abnormal metabolic processes of one kind or another.

- *Metabolic alkalosis* – indicated by a high bicarbonate (> 26 mmol/l) – is the least common acid–base abnormality. It might be due to there being fewer hydrogen ions than normal to buffer (e.g. because acid is being lost due to vomiting or large volumes of drainage from a nasogastric tube). Everything else being equal, a raised bicarbonate will increase blood pH.
- *Metabolic acidosis* is very common in acute and critical illness. It is indicated by low bicarbonate (< 22 mmol/l), and, everything else being equal, a decreased pH.

Renal failure

One cause of metabolic acidosis is renal failure, when there may be inadequate elimination of hydrogen ions by the kidneys, and/or reduced reabsorption of bicarbonate. Altered electrolyte balance also plays a part.

Ketoacidosis

Another cause of metabolic acidosis is ketoacidosis. This may occur in patients with poorly controlled diabetes mellitus, where fat rather than carbohydrate is being used as the body's main source of energy and ketones are produced as a by-product. Ketones form a strong acid, seen most strikingly in cases of diabetic ketoacidosis (DKA), when bicarbonate and pH levels may be extremely low. These patients often hyperventilate – and therefore have a low pCO_2 too. This is another example of a compensatory process: the individual cannot halt the production of ketones – and acid – without insulin, so they eliminate as much CO_2 as possible by breathing fast so that at least one potential source of acid is minimised.

Tissue hypoxia

The most common cause of metabolic acidosis in acute and critical illness is probably insufficient oxygen delivery to the tissues, because blood flow and/or blood pressure are too low, or because the patient is anaemic, or there simply is not enough oxygen in the blood. Tissue hypoxia changes the mechanisms of metabolism, and tends to increase the production of acid waste products, particularly lactic acid. Therefore, it is useful – if possible – to determine serum lactate in patients with metabolic acidosis, especially if there are signs or symptoms of circulatory failure. Some blood gas analyser machines are able to measure lactate levels in arterial blood samples, or a sample of venous blood in a grey topped sodium fluoride bottle may be sent to the laboratory. Hyperlactatemia (lactate > 3 mmol/l) is a marker of inadequate tissue oxygenation.

Poisoning and drugs

Many substances taken as poisons, either intentionally or accidentally (e.g. alcohol), and many medicines, prescribed or not (e.g. aspirin (salicylic *acid*)), can alter acid–base balance. Excessive administration of normal saline (sodium chloride 0.9%) solutions can cause hyperchloraemic acidosis.

Drugs that affect kidney function may contribute to either acidosis or alkalosis, depending on their specific action. Therefore, if an acid–base abnormality is present, the patient history and medications should also be reviewed.

Arterial blood gas analysis: summary

A simple, practical approach has been set out by the Resuscitation Council UK (2006).

1. Is the patient hypoxaemic? That is, is the pO_2 < 8 kPa (or SaO_2 < 90%)?

Arterial blood gas analysis: summary (cont'd)

- Consider the effects of oxygen therapy. If the patient requires more than 35% oxygen therapy to achieve a normal pO_2 and SaO_2, there is some acute or chronic disease process restricting the movement of oxygen into the circulatory system. Such a patient is at risk of further deterioration.

2. What is the pH?
   - pH > 7.45 = alkalaemia
   - pH < 7.35 = acidaemia.

3. What is the respiratory component?
   - pCO_2 > 6.1 kPa = respiratory acidosis (due to hypoventilation)
   - pCO_2 < 4.6 kPa = respiratory alkalosis (due to hyperventilation).

4. What is the metabolic component?
   - HCO_3^- < 22 mmol/l = metabolic acidosis
   - HCO_3^- < 26 mmol l = metabolic alkalosis.
   - Causes of metabolic acid–base disturbance include tissue hypoxia due to circulatory failure (leading to acidosis), renal dysfunction (usually acidosis, but sometimes alkalosis), ketoacidosis, and gastrointestinal losses (effects vary depending on whether the losses are from the stomach or lower gastrointestinal tract). Poisoning or medicines may also be a factor.

5. Was the HCO_3^- or pCO_2 abnormal? If so, look at the pH again.
   - If the HCO_3^- and pCO_2 are abnormal, but the pH is in the normal range, the abnormal HCO_3^- is being compensated by an abnormal pCO_2, or vice versa. As a rule of thumb, if the pH is < 7.4, it is most likely that the primary problem is that which is tending to make the blood more acid (i.e. a high pCO_2 or low HCO_3^-). If the pH is > 7.4, it is more likely that the primary problem is that which is tending to make the blood more alkali (i.e. a low pCO_2 or high HCO_3^-).

REFERENCE

Resuscitation Council UK (2006) Advanced Life Support (5th edn). Resuscitation Council UK, London

Appendix 2: Oxygen Delivery Devices

Commonly used oxygen administration devices, flow rates and approximate oxygen concentrations associated with those flow rates are shown below. It is not possible to determine precisely the exact concentration delivered by a particular flow rate through nasal cannulae, standard facemasks, or the high concentration mask shown here. This is because even patients breathing normally – and especially those breathing rapidly or deeply – inhale much larger volumes of air than can be supplied by a standard oxygen flowmeter, even when it is set to its maximum flow rate (usually 15 l/minute).

The average man in England weighs about 83 kg (Information Centre, 2006). Typically, breath volumes are 7 ml/kg bodyweight, so each of the average man's breaths are about 580 ml in size. With a respiratory rate of, say, 16, the average man has to take in almost 9.3 l per minute. But, inspiration occurs in about one-third of the respiratory cycle (as the remainder of the time is for expiration and a brief rest between breaths). Therefore, the man is actually required to take in all of the 9.3 l in one-third of a minute, meaning that average inspiratory flow to the lungs is 27.9 l/min. Even if the man is receiving oxygen at a flow of 15 l/min through a standard facemask, another 12.9 l of gas has to come from another source – that is, room air, which will dilute the oxygen. If he breathes rapidly or deeply – as is usually the case in respiratory failure – even more air will be taken in, and the oxygen further diluted.

NB: If the patient has a low oxygen saturation despite receiving high-concentration oxygen, one potential solution in the short term is to use a second source of oxygen and nasal cannulae to give 6 l oxygen through the nose as well as 15 l via a facemask.

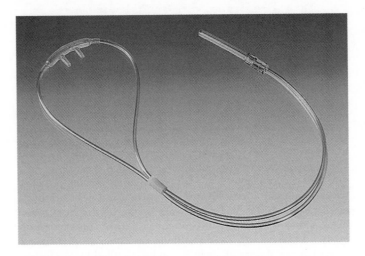

Reproduced with permission from Air Products Healthcare

Nasal cannulae

- O_2 flow 2–4 l/min (≤ 6 l for short periods)
- Precise regulation of O_2 concentration not possible

$$2 \, l/min \cong 28\% \; O_2$$
$$4 \, l/min \cong 36\% \; O_2$$

- Comfortable, allows patient to eat, drink, talk
- Nasal care may be needed due to drying effects.

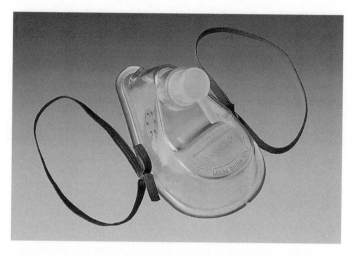

Reproduced with permission from Air Products Healthcare

'Standard' facemask/MC mask/Hudson mask

- O_2 flow $\geq$ 5–15 l/min
- Precise regulation of O_2 concentration not possible

$$5\,l/min \cong 35\%\ O_2$$
$$6\,l/min \cong 40\%\ O_2$$
$$8\,l/min \cong 50\%\ O_2$$

- Humidification is advisable if high-flow oxygen is being given for over 24 hours, or if the patient has thick and sticky secretions

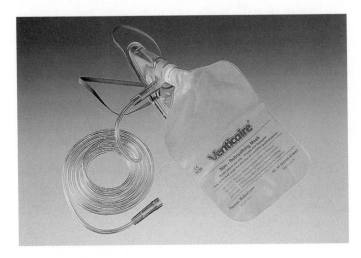

Reproduced with permission from Air Products Healthcare

High concentration mask with non-rebreathe reservoir bag

- O_2 flow $\geq$ 10–15 l/min
- Non-rebreathe reservoir bag should be inflated before applying to patient
- Precise regulation of O_2 concentration not possible

High flow device
Minimum flow = 10 l/min = approximately 85% O_2

- Cannot be humidified
- *Indicates the patient is at high-risk*

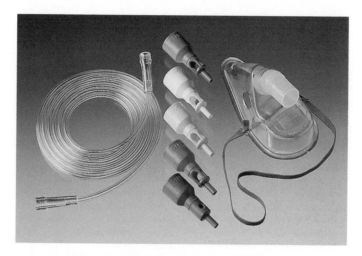

Reproduced with permission from Air Products Healthcare

Venturi mask

- O_2 flow 2–15 l/min, depending on which valve used
- Precise regulation of O_2 concentration is possible, e.g.,

> blue valve at 2 l/min = 24% O_2
> white valve at 4 l/min = 28% O_2
> orange valve at 6 l/min = 31% O_2
> yellow valve at 8 l/min = 35% O_2
> red valve at 10 l/min = 40% O_2

- Useful if risk of hypercapnic respiratory failure (e.g. chronic obstructive pulmonary disease)

REFERENCE

Information Centre (2006) Health Survey for England 2005 Latest Trends (Tables). NHS Information Centre (www.ic.nhs.uk/statistics-and-data-collections/healthand-lifestyles-related-surveys/health-survey-for-england/health-survey-for-england-2005-latest-trends)

Index